i ON BEAUTY

Endorsements

My husband Robert Wagner and I had the pleasure of meeting Irene shortly after she married our friend Arny Granat. We were immediately taken by Irene's spirit and beauty. She and I share much of the same philosophy about aging and life, also horses and dogs. Her well thought out and meticulously researched book is a must for those reaching what used to be called "a woman of a certain age". One look at Irene dispels that term completely. Thanks to Irene, This book tells us how to experience aging and how to be the best that you can be. What woman could ask for more?

JILL ST. JOHN,
Actress, Cookbook Author & Food Columnist

"Irene Michaels has written a breezy, readable, highly useful book about her own experiences and learnings regarding beauty—on the inside and out. Her spirit comes through on every page, as does the diligence with which she has been a lifelong learner regarding health and wellness. Irene has appreciated longer than most the connection between what you put in your body and what you put on your body, and readers will come away better informed and energized about how to live and be their best selves."

CHRISTIE HEFNER,
Chairman, Hatchbeauty Brands, former Executive Chairman, Canyon Ranch Enterprises, former Chairman/ CEO Playboy Enterprises

"Irene Michaels has rapidly become a trusted name in the beauty and luxury lifestyle industries as her skincare products have revolutionized the anti-aging world. I'm proud to call her a dear friend, and could not be more excited for her (and all of us who gain from her wisdom) as she publishes her extraordinary debut book, *I On Beauty*."

RITA COSBY,
Emmy-Winning TV Host & Best Selling Author

"Irene Michaels' debut book, *I On Beauty*, Living Beautifully and Luxuriously Beyond 50, embodies that 50 is the BEGINNING, not the END! This book is Fabulous!!"

NIKKI HASKELL,
Pop Culture Historian & Creator of
Star Shooterz

I'm not sure if there's a better book for women over 50 looking to improve their skincare routine and cosmetic health. Not only is everything scientifically backed, but it's also completely safe. Looking your best as the years add up may sound daunting, but trust me, it couldn't be simpler thanks to Irene. Her expertise in beauty as a model and actress remains, and it's a wonder why she took all this time to finally write a book.

MARGAUX LEVY,
Attorney & Creator of Skincare Brands: Freeze 24*7®,
Reversital® & Unline™ Originals

i ON BEAUTY

LIVING BEAUTIFULLY & LUXURIOUSLY BEYOND 50

IRENE MICHAELS

Beauty & Luxury Lifestyle Expert

Published by Best Seller Publishing®, Pasadena, CA
Best Seller Publishing® is a registered trademark
Printed in the United States of America.
ISBN _____

This publication is designed to provide accurate and authoritative information with regard to the subject matter covered. It is sold with the understanding that the publisher is not engaged in rendering legal, accounting, or other professional advice. If legal advice or other expert assistance is required, the services of a competent professional should be sought. The opinions expressed by the authors in this book are not endorsed by Best Seller Publishing® and are the sole responsibility of the author rendering the opinion.

For more information, please write:
Best Seller Publishing®
253 N. San Gabriel Blvd, Unit B
Pasadena, CA 91107
or call 1(626) 765 9750
Visit us online at: www.BestSellerPublishing.org

Table of Contents

TO MY MOTHER,
A BEAUTY INSIDE & OUT

I will be Forever grateful for the warmth, grace
and love you showed me my entire life.
You taught me how to love, forgive, accept and always
have hope through life's trials and tribulations.
I will always love you.
See you on the other side.

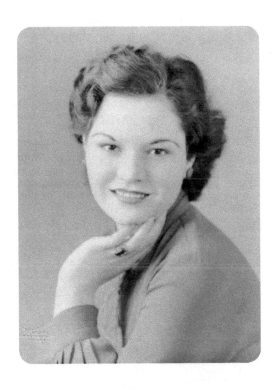

SPECIAL THANKS

A huge thank you to Suzanne Tripaldi,
for her dedication and passion in helping
me write this book.

Foreword

BY

Dr. Robert A. Goldman MD, DO, PhD, FAASP

Co-Founder/Chairman-A4M American
Academy of Anti-Aging Medicine

While aging provides exciting new adventures and opportunities, it also brings seemingly endless detriments to our health and beauty. Reaching 50 can mean more time with the children, newfound hobbies, and hopefully a sense of security as retirement approaches. But it also spawns a whole new problem, one that compounds from a lifetime of work and stress: wrinkles.

My name is Dr. Robert Goldman, and I have lived my life as a martial artist, world-champion athlete, and philanthropist. As the Co-founder of the American Academy of Anti-Aging Medicine, World Anti-Aging Academy of Medicine, and The International Sports Hall of Fame, I've focused much of my energy on the world of anti-aging through medicine and science. Not only that, but I'm over 50 myself!

Through my experience in the field of anti-aging medicine, I have discovered that people will do almost anything to appear younger than they really are. Ridiculous gimmicks found behind click-bait ads and infomercials are par for the course, but the solution doesn't have to be so complex. The first steps to maintaining glorious skin as the years add up are debunking the common myths surrounding aging, something that this book does extraordinary well.

I On Beauty - *Living Beautifully and Luxuriously Beyond 50.* is a groundbreaking book in the world of health, beauty & anti-aging. Blending traditional methods with modern twists, Irene has created an encyclopedia for beauty after 50. She begins by putting common misconceptions to bed and follows them up with simple tips to maintain skin health. No tricks or gimmicks, just methods proven for smoother skin. Irene has also laid out a skincare plan with better habits to incorporate into your routine and provides tips for a healthier diet and healthier hair.

Irene Michaels has become a trusted name in the beauty industry. I'm proud to call her a close friend, and could not be more excited for her as she publishes her debut book, I On Beauty - *Living Beautifully and Luxuriously Beyond 50.*

This is an excellent book for women over 50 looking to improve their skincare routine and cosmetic health. Not only is it scientifically backed, but it is also safe. Looking your best as the years add up may sound daunting, but trust me, it couldn't be simpler thanks to Irene. Her expertise in beauty as a model and actress remains, and it's a wonder why she took all this time to finally write a book.

I highly recommend I On Beauty - *Living Beautifully and Luxuriously Beyond 50* for those approaching or over the age of fifty. In today's day and age, stress is at an all-time high and aging may be on the back burner of our minds. Thankfully, Irene has even included a section solely dedicated to cosmetic health in our COVID-19 world.

Now, without further ado, dive into the book and see for yourself the amazing benefits within.

Introduction

When I was a little girl, I would sit on my front porch watching my neighbors pass by, and I'd say, "Hi! What's your name?" And when I'd get my answer, I'd go on to inquire, "And what do you do?" I must have been six years old. My mother used to tell me, "Oh, you're going to be the next Ann Landers." Ann Landers, the syndicated advice columnist who appeared in newspapers across the country, was big at the time. And then, there were the many hours I spent on the phone as a young girl, listening to my friends' problems. My mother would say, "Irene, you've got to take all that creativity and compassion and put it to good use someday." And that is what I have done my entire life.

I feel that I have a lifetime of experience to share, starting from when I was a little girl. As a child, I was very inquisitive and creative, and I loved playing make-believe. I was curious and adventurous, and I have stayed that way my whole life. And so, I have been contemplating writing a book for some time now, and I am so happy that, at last, the time to do so has arrived.

My cousin, Cathy, was very creative as well, and when I was in middle school, she invited me to come along to one of her dance lessons. Now that was something I had no idea about. But I was ready to give it a try. My mother bought me tap shoes, and together we took a bus to the studio. And I started taking tap lessons. I had no idea of what I was doing, but on that first day, I fell in love with dance. So I started taking lessons along with my cousin, and long after she had stopped, I continued on. Actually, I still take tap lessons.

What I learned in those early lessons was that I have dancing in my blood. I've wanted to be a dancer ever since, and I have spent much time learning and studying dance. One time, as I was doing some exploring, I met a woman by the name of Claire Powell. Claire owned a studio in the city of Chicago called Powell Academy for the Arts. I came from humble beginnings, but I knew one thing: I wanted to take a bunch of classes and become a professional dancer.

Whenever I could afford it, I would go to Claire's studio after school and take classes, paying for them with money in an envelope, or even in coins, whichever I happened to have available. She felt that I had something and was so impressed that, after a while, she took me under her wing and made me her protégé, paying for all my training. For the next decade, she taught me, I learned, and I went on tour with a young dance group. We worked in state fairs and all kinds of parties, private parties for prominent people. Claire said that

I had that sparkle, and I believed her. So I kept on studying. Eventually, I ended up in an off-Broadway production, and I kept on dancing. But as we all know, a dancer's life as a dancer is short.

At thirty years of age, a dancer is generally considered washed up. I did some dancing until I was almost forty. So I was very, very lucky. In my twenties, I was asked to do a modeling gig. I knew nothing about modeling. So of course, I said, "I'd better take this opportunity."

In fact, I jumped at that opportunity, and in a short time, maybe one year or so, I became one of the top ten models in Chicago. I was in several local magazines, and I won several beauty contests. I was given the title of Miss Photoflash in the first such contest I ever won.

Over time, in moving forward from dancing and modeling, at age twenty-seven, I decided to open my own modeling agency. Within one year of opening, I had around thirty-nine employees. I specialized in fashion shows, and I was on a pretty good roll. And then, at the height of my career, something horrible happened. One day, I was thrown through a car windshield in an auto accident, shattering the entire left side of my face.

Never Defeated

I sustained a blowout fracture in my eye, along with acquiring 1500 stitches. There went my beloved modeling career. It took me over three years to get better and regain my confidence. It was a great deal of work and a big challenge and a very sad time for me. However, by the end of three years, I refused to be defeated.

Hitting the ground running, I turned my interest to music. I always was fascinated by all aspects of the arts, whether dancing, acting, modeling, and now music. I loved any artistic form of expression. At that time, I started guitar lessons, and I still take them today. Within six months, I was also singing and taking a few acting lessons. And I had an audition in Los Angeles!

A friend had submitted a photograph of me from my modeling days because a studio was auditioning for a role on "General Hospital." It was quite a popular TV soap opera at the time. I flew to LA, I did the audition, and lo and behold, I got the role, which just happened to be a recurring role as a nurse. I was so fortunate, and I moved to LA and stayed there for a few years.

I was living with one of the stars of "General Hospital" in her coach house, and that was quite an experience. On my right side, was Bob Hope. On my left, Alice Cooper, practicing his guillotine act. And then, across the street, was Sally Field. As I said, quite an experience!

My landlady used to smoke marijuana with her toes. And I thought, "Well, how interesting is that?"

To say the least, it was indeed an interesting time for me. I learned so many tricks of the trade during that period. My face was still not right due to the damage incurred in the accident. Even so, I was on "General Hospital." I learned to stay away from certain angles, and I did a lot of research on certain makeups to find ways to cover my scars. It took me probably a good five or six years to find the right combination.

Over the years, I appeared in several feature films and on stage in various theater productions. My career later shifted from working in front of the camera to behind the camera as an entrepreneur and producer. I formed two production companies that produced promotional events for corporations, hotels, and convention centers. I built the Showtime modeling agency from the ground up and managed to keep it running flawlessly for over two decades. Eventually, this is the path I took—to become a Beauty and Luxury Lifestyle Expert.

As time passed, I decided to write. I was getting older and had met a lot of challenges in my life. I had experienced so many life lessons—in beauty, glamour, tragedy, and back. I wasn't acting on camera or doing much dancing any longer, or not even much modeling. So I decided it was time to chronicle my experiences.

One of the peak moments in my career began when I created my signature brand, "I On ... " The first use of my brand was for my website, which directly led to numerous opportunities, including a cover story for Resident Magazine. (To read the full article go to: https://issuu.com/ resident_mag/docs/__issuu_jan_2019_irene_michaels/100) My website, "I On The Scene" https://ionthescene.com (the I, of course, stands for *Irene*), which I started in 2008, has become a high-traffic website focusing on beauty and luxury lifestyles. Considered an authority site, as of the time of this book's publication, it has grown to over 15,000 daily users, over 450,000 users per month with multiple page views per visit, with more than fifty contributors and over 750 posts.

"BE PART OF THE SCENE." Want to know about upcoming events, features, giveaways and more? Sign up for our newsletter and never miss a beat.

Sign up here: (https://ionthescene.com/sign-up/)

It was only a matter of time. With my beauty experience and background, with all the tricks of the trade that I'd acquired in covering my scars, and with all the celebrities I had met, I decided maybe I'd just develop my anti-aging skincare line with Suzanne. After consulting with a beauty industry icon, we started my product line, which we called I On Youth Collection by Irene Michaels™. We all want to be youthful. I want to be youthful, so it worked for me. *How perfect*, I thought, *I On Youth.*

I felt that I had something real to share with other women. Because of what had happened to me, I wanted to share my story, and let women know that no matter what you feel, no matter how depressed you may be, no matter what things have happened to you, you need never feel defeated.

It's the Journey That Matters

Always remember that the longest road starts with the first step. And it is not what happens to you, it is how you handle it! Determination is key. I never let anything stop me from being my very best. I am always conscious of that. I am also aware of how fear can enter your life, and it can immobilize any of us. It is a big deal, so you have to be careful about that. It is not an easy task, but if you work at it, you can overcome it. That is where your meditation practice and your beliefs and your faith come in.

If I were to tell someone today that I had these fears, that I was very self-conscious, and that I felt ugly, that person would have a good laugh. They would look at me and say, "You, this outgoing, mature, gorgeous creature—you must have been born with a silver spoon in your mouth." Boy, nothing could be further from the truth. But to sum it all up: I had a dream. I never give up, despite any downfalls. Any rocky road one travels is a long road. But it is the journey that matters. Love yourself. And be kind.

This book is meant for women over fifty. A mature audience, one that is interested in staying healthy and young, in looking good, in feeling vibrant and sexy. You need a little vanity. You must take care of yourself, no matter what. In this book, I want to continue to explore and explain and share with women my extensive life experiences, including coming back from a very bad accident.

Let me say this to start with—it is not horrible to get old! What matters is not only your beauty outside but even more so, your beauty inside. Beauty is not skin deep—it comes from within. You have to have a healthy attitude, and that all begins with loving yourself. My dedication is to stay healthy, inside and out, and to look good as long as I can.

I guess my biggest fear is not being able to take care of myself, to become disabled in some way, and not able to continue my disciplines and regimens that I love so much. I know how frustrating it is to watch your skin sag, your belly drop, and your eyes start in with the wrinkles. The whiteness of your eyes disappears, and your energy is no more. The pains that occur, day in and day out, I do know all of that. But you have faith, you have courage.

Sustaining hair loss, not being able to wear high heels, I know how that may sound silly to some, but it can feel important to us women. We want to feel glamorous, no matter what. We want to feel sexy and desired by the other gender, and sometimes as we get older, we don't feel sexy any longer. But there are ways to help us keep on feeling some of that sizzle. Put on a beautiful dress. Put on your high heels and get yourself made up. Go for it.

You will find much in this book to help you feel sexy and glamorous and attractive. The chapters that follow cover myths of aging, anti-aging secrets, skin habits, and great food for your skin as it ages. You'll find do-it-yourself, straight-from-your-kitchen haircare, beyond-sixty styles and tips, and insights on makeup for skin and eyes as well as maintaining your kit. And I will tell you all about how my life is made even more joyful with animals, all my wonderful furry friends. All my animals that I love enrich my life and help keep me giving and compassionate every day. And then, there are a few words on living through this time of COVID-19.

I hope you enjoy this book, as well as feel more prepared and fabulously confident once you have read it. Moving through middle-age and getting older is not the end of life. It is wonderful. Keep motivated. Keep engaged. You'll be, well, just like my name—*Irene:*

> **I** *will,*
>
> **R**ewire not retire,
>
> **E**ngage,
>
> **N**ever give up, and
>
> **E**ndure.

50 is the BEGINNING, not the END

CHAPTER 1

Myths of Aging

It is only recently that I've started feeling my age. I think that more demands in regard to aging are put on a person—woman or man—in the entertainment world. It is not as easy sometimes to age gracefully when living so much in the public eye. What they say is, as you get older, you get a different ache and pain every day. Well, that's true. I have had a good run for a very long time of feeling and looking good. But I realize I'm not young anymore, per se. It's been coming on little by little, I guess. But it does seem so sudden, when a variety of small signs all seem to pop up and make you realize, you're just there.

I remember a friend of mine saying something to me years ago. I was younger than my friend, who was about forty-three. We'd talk about age, and in my opinion, she was still young. But she said, "I just feel horrible getting old."

"Well, I don't think you're so old," I told her. "What makes you feel that way?"

And then she said, "You know what I've noticed? None of the guys look at me anymore. No men find me attractive. I don't feel sexy, and it makes me sad."

My friend's viewpoint has not been my experience. Most times, people will say something like, "God! I thought you were fifty. You look so young." In reality, if you were to assess how youthful is the appearance of a person of sixty, seventy, or seventy-five when standing next to a real fifty-year-old, there's no contest. After sixty, you simply do not look like that. But it is nice to hear.

The Biggest Myths about Women & Aging

Aging is a biological process of becoming older. Since aging is a natural and inevitable phenomenon, you'd expect it would be welcomed with open arms. Quite the opposite in recent times. Aging for so many people is met with mixed feelings and perceptions. We can blame social media and our society in general for this negative vision of aging. However, it is important to know that how you respond to such trends is a personal choice.

Today, most people have embraced the concept of aging as a bad thing, something to be hidden. Others just want to avoid whatever symptoms they can, continuing to live their normal lives whilst enjoying smooth, radiant skin.

As a result of this more modern concept of aging, particularly as it relates to women, several pervasive myths on the topic are being spread and passed for facts. These myths have women of all ages on their toes.

MYTH 1: Women do not like to reveal their age: Some people believe that most women are ashamed of their age, especially older women. Research has found this to be untrue and applicable to only a small percentage of women. Most women are open to disclosing their age to people of any gender. The few who choose to hide it do so out of insecurity rather than the fear of aging.

MYTH 2: All women use anti-aging creams or solutions: Not all women use anti-aging creams. Some women may use them to reduce the appearance of wrinkles, while others opt for different methods like sheet masques. Other women use none of these.

MYTH 3: SPF is important for the face alone: SPF should be applied on the neck as well as the face. If used on only the face, the skin of the neck might age at a more rapid rate than the facial skin. But by the time you reach your fifties, the skin of each could end up looking severely different. Start the safe process now.

MYTH 4: Aging means losing your fashion sense: This is untrue. Women (and men alike) are not being held back by age when it comes to fashion. They continue to dress as they desire, regardless of age.

MYTH 5: Wrinkles are the most important sign of aging: This is untrue. So much about this topic is misunderstood. Wrinkles can appear when a person undergoes stress for a period of time. Research has also proven that wrinkles can be hereditary in some people. And while wrinkles are a sign of aging, they are not the most important or obvious one. Myths such as these distract women from the true signs of aging: sunken cheeks and under-eye hollowing. These signs can start to develop soon after reaching forty.

MYTH 6: You need more foundation as you age: Heavier layers of foundation will only harden the face, making you look even older. When age creeps in, it is time to use less foundation and invest more in tinted moisturizers.

MYTH 7: Using makeup with SPF is adequate protection: The sun inflicts significant harmful effects on the skin of the face, which is why SPF should be an important part of your daily life. Using makeup with a level of SPF is not going to give you the protection you need, unless you intend to use up the entire product in an application. Apply a small amount of sunscreen each day. You'll protect your skin from the damaging effects of the sun, while allowing the enzymes to work toward healing.

MYTH 8: An effective moisturizer can fight wrinkles: This is quite misunderstood. A moisturizer does not lessen wrinkles, rather the water within them is what hydrates the skin to reduce wrinkles.

MYTH 9: Aging depends on genes in women: Genes play a small but significant role in aging for each gender. However, other factors such as pollution, sun, lifestyle, and smoking contribute as much as 90 percent to signs of aging.

MYTH 10: Expensive anti-aging products are the most effective: This is false. The high cost of an anti-aging product does not guarantee its effectiveness. Most quality products are affordable and easily available. Look for those with the right active ingredients.

MYTH 11: Diet does not influence aging: Diet influences aging. Foods with a high glycemic index can accelerate aging and contribute to sagging skin. They may also make the skin vulnerable and susceptible to the damaging effects of the sun. Such foods include bread, potatoes, pasta, and so on.

MYTH 12: Sunscreen is unimportant on a cloudy day: This myth suggests that UV rays may not be present on cloudy days. It is a wrong assumption as UV rays are present all year round, each day. It occurs in smaller doses that pass through the clouds, causing hyperpigmentation and elastin breakdown. Therefore, sunscreen is important every day you are out of the house. And that is not restricted to just women or those that are older.

Still Modeling after 70

Do you find that hard to believe? Well, it's true! Throughout my life, I have worn many hats, and the most lucrative has been modeling. As some of you may know, most modeling careers are over by the age of forty. I believe one of the reasons my career has lasted so long is my attitude and zest for life. For example, since I never could decide which art I loved the most, I took up all of them! I have spent my life practicing dancing, acting, modeling, playing guitar, singing, boxing, and horseback riding . . . and the list goes on.

During my life, I have had much success as a lifestyle model, and I'm happy to say, I have also enjoyed the pleasures of being an experienced equestrian. This skill has enabled me to compete in show jumping across the United States as well as internationally. I also cover international horse events for I On The Scene. A favorite event of mine was in 2016 in England: Riding Weekend Burley Manor in New Forest National Park, Hampshire—it was a wonderful weekend!

I remember as a young woman, my mother would have preferred for me to be a homemaker. At the same time, my father was encouraging me to see the world. That is what I did! Throughout my journey, I have encountered so many wonderful people, talented artists, and other great models, all while visiting parts of the world that I had only dreamed of.

Many times, I am asked how I still have the energy to juggle traveling, modeling, and being married to my wonderful husband, Arny, as well as fulfilling social obligations, continuing lessons, and engaging in endless hours of maintenance. The answer is, "It ain't easy," and anyone who tells you that it is, is lying.

As we age, our regimen gets more involved, requiring more effort, especially in the modeling industry. You have to stay on top of current fashions and the newest beauty and makeup trends. There is also the endless battle to stay thin, not to mention finding the right skin care, staying on top of the proper diet, and making it all seem effortless.

Being in the industry, I have learned many beauty secrets, dozens of shortcuts, and great sources to help a person stay young. Yet, after trying so many brands that simply didn't work, I decided to develop my own anti-aging skincare line—I On Youth Collection by Irene Michaels™.

I would have to say that one of the types of jobs I dislike the most is when I get a call to audition for a product like Depends. I look in the mirror and say to myself, "Am I that old?!" Yep, I guess I am. However, there's the other side of the coin—in the same week as such an audition, I'll also be asked to go on a cruise ship and model cruise wear on an island somewhere. So, like anything in life, there comes a point where you have to adjust. And it does not hurt to have wonderful representation.

A funny thing happened one day when I was sitting in a doctor's office. When the nurse called my name to go in for my appointment, she said, "I saw you sitting there for a long time, but I thought for sure that the woman I was looking for must have left. When I saw the age on the card, I thought,

'It can't be her!'" Finally, she came up and asked me, and she just could not believe that I was the older woman.

The nurse went on to say that I looked like a forty-year-old, not seventy-one. I replied, "Yes, until you stand me next to a real forty-year-old. There is no escaping time."

I believe it is a luxury to grow older. Of course, we all want to look twenty-seven forever, but if you can allow yourself to age gracefully, appreciating all you have, spirit will keep you young. Believe it or not, it is more difficult for a man to enter midlife than for a woman. Men today dye and streak their hair, get injected with Botox and other fillers, get liposuction and plastic surgery. Truly, they are vainer than women.

The whole aging process is interesting to me. I believe you should simply be who you are, feeling the strength and power you possess as a beautiful human being. That will shine through brighter than any highlighter.

Remember, you can be anything and do anything with a strong desire and the approval you give yourself to believe that it's okay to be older. That, along with much dedication, discipline, and belief in yourself can help you accomplish great things at any age.

Need proof? I'm still modeling after seventy. Just sayin'!

Seven Anti-Aging Tips to Flawless Skin

Who does not enjoy the sweet remembrance of those days when we were young, free and easy, living without the stress of fine lines and wrinkles on the skin?

Adopting methods and approaches that promise to make a person appear much younger than their age has become a familiar ideal. Many techniques—natural and artificial—can be used to make yourself look like you are living in the good, old (and young) days. Some individuals opt for anti-aging treatments such as Botox or other surgical treatments, and yet do not achieve the desired results.

I believe you will find that natural methods are the better way to acquire the anti-aging phenomenon. Though achieving that outcome may seem relatively slow, these methods are less harmful than the artificial techniques available. And natural methods provide a lasting result. Here are a few of my favorite natural anti-aging secrets to enjoy flawless skin:

1 – USE A MILD CLEANSER FOR WASHING YOUR SKIN

Cleansing is an essential part of your daily routine as it helps to achieve a healthier and younger look. It is the basic step for individuals who work outdoors and are subject to allergies and dust, and who perform makeup regularly. Use cleansers that are gentle on your skin and do not result in dehydration or a moisture-stripping effect. Select cleansers with low pH and avoid buying cleansers with sodium lauryl sulphate.

2 – USE A SUITABLE TONER

People harbor the misconception that toner is not an essential part of the everyday skin routine. However, the truth of the matter is the opposite. Toner is as essential as the right cleaners. Use toners in your daily routine after cleansing because they help maintain your skin pH.

3 – EXFOLIATE

Exfoliation is an important part of your daily routine. Dermatologists have recommended for years that exfoliation not be performed on a daily basis. However, in modern times, dermatologists now believe that exfoliation should be performed every day to achieve proper cleaning by removing the outer layers. Use a scrub with fine crystals and avoid the ones that use abrasions or micro-cuts.

4 – MOISTURIZE

Celebrities and dermatologists swear by achieving truly vibrant skin using various anti-aging skincare options, which, of course, involve use of a moisturizer. Apply the moisturizer to your skin after it is perfectly exfoliated. Use a gentle, upward motion so that it absorbs completely into your skin. Use an appropriate moisturizer, chosen according to your age and skin type.

5 – EAT A VEGAN DIET

Incorporate healthy foods into your diet to maintain flawless and young skin. Consume foods rich in vitamin C, antioxidants, beta carotene, vitamin A, and vitamin E such as berries, oranges, sweet potatoes, carrots, spinach, whole grains, almonds, and others.

Avoid consumption of processed sugar as it breaks down and causes the loss of elastin and collagen fibers in your body, resulting in sagging skin and the formation of wrinkles.

6 – PRACTICE MEDITATION

Meditation is key to achieving a flawless and younger look. Meditation allows the skin to inhale oxygen leading to new cell formation. Regeneration of cells results in a younger and brighter look.

7 – SLEEP

Taking a deep and restful sleep for at least seven to eight hours daily naturally keeps your skin healthier. Sleep deprivation results in sagging, puffy eyes and wrinkle formation over the skin. Sleeping well at night results in the formation of growth hormones, which allows the regeneration of new skin cells.

Stress is the key factor that results in aging. Avoiding the aged look requires regular self-care to mitigate the effects of stress in the form of performing meditation, exercising, eating healthy fruits and vegetables, keeping yourself hydrated, and performing regular *cleaning, toning,* and *moisturizing* (CTM) in your daily skincare routine.

If you are looking for more options, there are other anti-aging treatments you could consider (such as peptides), which have an effect in reversing the aging process.

Accepting Yourself Where You Are

In my own personal journey in life, there has been no middle. I always felt like I was jumping from one phase to the next, with no in-betweens. Kindergarten to high school, college to the stage, one big jump after another, so that I never felt like I was just living through those interim periods. So when it comes to this in-between time of aging, it can feel a bit overwhelming.

Thinking about it, there have been little signs right along, signaling change. For instance, I can't get on my horse as easily as I used to. I remember a time last year when I wanted to go for a bike ride. And I'll be darned, I couldn't get my leg over the seat. That was eye-opening. And I started noticing I couldn't walk quite as far as I used to, and I'm a pretty good walker. I'd always taken long walks, so it just didn't make sense to me.

I rarely get bored, but sometimes if I do, I'll start cleaning my kitchen cabinets. I may do something silly like take everything out of my closet and organize, standing on my chair as needed to get to the upper back shelf. Well, not long ago, I gave that a try and found I couldn't raise my body after stepping on the chair. *Well now, that is strange*, I thought. But I didn't give it much more thought. Not until I found out from my doctor that I needed a total hip replacement. Another sign of aging. But I will be back dancing as soon as I can.

As I mentioned in the introduction, and I've said it many times, *it's not what happens to you, it's how you handle it.* So here's a tip: If you want to feel younger, hang around with younger people. Too many times, when you get on the phone and chat with older friends, all you hear about are their aches and pains. Their headache, their nose ache, their elbow ache, their back ache. You name it, they have it. So you can see why I think it may be better to try to be with someone a little younger. They can simply be more fun to be around, and maybe not so inclined to just complain about life, making you feel a little younger as well.

That's why men date younger women. Whenever I would see a couple like that, I'd wonder, "What do they have in common?" Well, one thing that they do not have in common is all the aches and pains and BS that so many older women have. The baggage, the kids, the problems, financial pressures—when you're young, you don't have that kind of baggage. It doesn't mean you don't have any baggage when you're young; it's just different.

You can make it harder on yourself, if you do not accept your own aging. It is too easy to let yourself fall into a rut. Young or old, it is just a matter of living your life—but you need to look at the happier side of life. Always stay positive, always be feeling something positive. If you find yourself getting pulled into a negative thought, replace it in with a positive one. That is what will pull you through.

CHAPTER 2

Anti-Aging Secrets & Tips

In Hollywood, a woman is considered on the older side at the age of thirty. Forty, no question about it. It's tough getting older in Hollywood. And it isn't about your age, in and of itself. It's about your skin. That, as we know, changes as you get older. Things start to sag. Your eyes are not quite as white as they once were. And the jobs are just not coming your way any longer.

Of course, we can all name the exceptions: Glenn Close, Meryl Streep, and Jane Fonda, for example. All true actresses, who have been working forever. Most women don't find themselves in that position. I suppose you could look at it like this: If you have a hot, new, flashy, sexy TV show going on, you wouldn't put a sixty-year-old in it as the star. They won't have the same energy as a young person, and audiences are pretty fickle.

I always looked young for my age, and so I wasn't feeling my age so much for most of my life. I was always too young to be old and too old to be young when it came to my modeling business. My discipline and regimen from early in my life of being a dancer, and then an actress and a model, taught me good habits and techniques. It felt very natural for me to just take good care of myself, a gift not everyone has the benefit of.

A lot of women do not have that discipline. But you can maintain discipline if you can get it started. And you'll find, once you are disciplined, if you let even a day go by, you feel horrible about it. It's a good practice, and if you at least try it, you may be surprised how fast it will come along.

My mother used to see me in my room getting ready and doing my face and hair, and she'd say, "Irene, I can't tell you how you drive me crazy. You look in the mirror and fluff a little powder on, a little eye pencil, some lipstick." In my mother's case, she didn't have any eyebrows, so it took her an hour to draw them on. I suppose she could have learned a different technique that was less time consuming, but things were very different for her back then.

Anyway, I attribute a lot of my discipline today to what I learned from my dancing days. Even today, if I can't do these things, I continually reinvent myself, and I'd like to say, in pretty grand style. It's amazing how fast the years fly by, and yet, when you are young, you never think of time. All of a sudden, as an older person, you look at every day like a ticking clock. You feel your own mortality, and you have to do something about it. You have to replace that feeling that came so easily during your youth. Perhaps that's why I dive into my music and some of the other things I do, so I don't let myself fall into feeling that way. I just have too much life to live to let that happen. Again, it comes down to replacing negativity with positivity.

Best Anti-Aging Secrets

We have been searching for the ultimate anti-aging tips and secrets throughout the ages, and in modern times, we look to the dermatologists or the hairdressers to find out their secrets. So, let's have a look at how to get the flawless skin with minimal pores we all desire, and to reduce signs of aging. Here are the best anti-aging tips and secrets:

MAKE USE OF SESAME OIL

Apply sesame oil in the morning all over your face and body. This oil is essential for proper blood circulation and hydration. It offers a glow to your skin while removing dead skin cells.

AVOID USING FOUNDATION

Using foundations on a regular basis results in more noticeable effects by showing off wrinkles and fine lines. A moisturizer with a dab of concealer is a far better choice for use on areas such as blemishes or under-eye circles.

FOLLOW A SIMPLE SKINCARE ROUTINE

If you are not in a position to indulge yourself in a seven- to ten-step skincare regimen, at a cost of several hundred dollars, even if only because it is not convenient, you may want to consider this advice. Follow a simple skincare regimen such as exfoliating, cleansing, using a toner for your skin type, and moisturizing with a product containing an SPF.

AVOID CONSUMPTION OF WHITE SUGAR

Processed sugar intake results in speeding up the aging process by weakening collagen fibers in the skin and contributing to premature formation of wrinkles with sagging skin. The better course would be to consume more vegetables and fruits instead of sugar, and use sugar for exfoliation only. When used for scrubbing the skin, sugar is great at helping to exfoliate it, effectively removing impurities and leaving a fresh complexion.

SLEEP WELL

Getting seven to eight hours of sleep each day and applying night creams over your eyes and face are essential routines. These are key secrets to keeping your face fresh and healthy with a glowing look, and your fine lines and wrinkles less visible.

HAVE A MASSAGE

Getting a massage from an expert helps in relieving stress and makes you feel young and energetic. A deep-tissue massage, and reflexology, in particular, offers a relaxing effect.

Gifts of Nature

Every one of us desires wrinkle-free skin with a perfect glow and an appearance of youthfulness. With age, we all start showing signs that are a natural part of the aging process, whether we like them or not, such as new creases and deepening facial lines. So, here are some natural anti-aging tips, which do not result in harmful effects to the skin:

CONSUME AN ANTI-INFLAMMATORY DIET AND SPICES

Cayenne pepper and turmeric are the two most commonly available and best anti-inflammatory spices. Adding these spices to your lunch and dinner meals will easily contribute to reversing the process of aging, as will adopting an anti-inflammatory diet overall. Add vegetables and monosaturated fats rich in omega-3, as well as avoid consumption of sugar and refined carbohydrates.

OZONATED OILS

Oxygen is an essential factor for reversing the aging process. Detox your skin, as well as your whole body, with the use of ozonated oils. These oils are fantastic skin moisturizers, helping to improve wrinkles, age spots, and fine lines. Ozonated oils also work well for mitigating eczema and helping to fight against infections.

ALOE VERA

Do not underestimate aloe vera, which is rich in essential minerals, vitamins, fatty acids, amino acids, and water. This plant serves as among the best of nature's gifts for hydration of the skin. This natural moisturizer increases the elasticity of the skin and helps in reducing wrinkles.

ANTI-AGING OXIDANTS

Start consuming anti-aging oxidants, which include vitamin E, C, and selenium. These serve as anti-inflammatory agents and are great at keeping skin healthy. The perfect antioxidants, they protect your skin against damage by UV radiation and promote collagen formation.

Get started with any of these recommended natural anti-aging tips for the wrinkle-free and glowing skin you love. Making some healthy alterations in your lifestyle such as improving your diet, doing the right amount and types of exercise, and creating a stress-free environment will all work wonders for sustaining youthful skin.

Active vs. Inactive Ingredients in Skincare

Have you ever really looked at the list of ingredients on the back label of a skincare product you picked up off the shelf in a store? Did you then feel confused and simply turn back to the front product label to see what was being said in simpler terms? Did you wonder what those confusing ingredients could mean or feel that some of them might have just as well been left out?

The good news is, you are not alone in your confusion. All these questions mean is that you want what everyone else wants—safe, healthy, and effective products!

Unfortunately, it's pretty difficult to tell what is safe and healthy anymore. Even organic products cannot be completely trusted. The best solution comes down to knowing what is on that ingredient list. Well, I can tell you this: There are two categories you need to be aware of—*active ingredients and inactive ingredients.*

You may have seen products that specify these categories and others that don't. Knowing what each of them imply can enhance your skincare product decision for the better.

What Are Active Ingredients?

An active ingredient is an ingredient meant to treat or address a condition. It is the ingredient that takes action and does what the product says it will do. An active ingredient is approved by the United States Food and Drug Administration (FDA) to perform a specific function.

An active ingredient for a skin product can fight inflammation, treat conditions, reverse photoaging, boost cell regeneration, and more. Here are some examples of active ingredients you may have come across: hydroquinone for skin lightening, titanium dioxide for sun protection, and benzoyl peroxide for acne.

What Are Inactive Ingredients?

What would be the opposite of active ingredients? Inactive ingredients do not provide any direct benefit in improving a condition or perform a specific function in that regard. However, they perform other equally important functions in completing the usefulness of a product. An inactive ingredient in a skincare product will do any of the following:

- **Stabilize:** Inactive ingredients act as stabilizers, maintaining the product's consistency and texture, and keeping it from degrading too quickly.
- **Transport:** Inactive ingredients can be used as carriers to deliver the active ingredients to their effective point of action. For this, most products use water.
- **Preserve:** Preventing contamination to the product or skin is a preservative function of inactive ingredients. (Parabens, which can be problematic, are an example of such ingredients.)
- **Enhance:** Inactive ingredients can make the product smell nice and look nice.

Where Active and Inactive Ingredients Meet

The fact that an ingredient is inactive does not mean it will have no effect on the skin. Ingredients come in contact with the skin and eventually find their way into the body. This is why some inactive ingredients are prohibited from use. Synthetic perfumes might sensitize the skin, serums with other inactive ingredients can irritate the skin, and parabens are known to play a role in breast cancer.

While the adverse effects of some inactive ingredients are a consideration, there is also the issue of balance in terms of the overall effectiveness of a product. Many brands reduce the number of active ingredients and increase the inactive ingredients that make you feel and smell good. So an active ingredient being listed on the label does not guarantee the product's effectiveness.

A Time for Everything

When the time came that I started to reveal my age in the public eye, my modeling agencies were not happy with me. They gave me a lot of flack over it. It began around the time of the birth of my serum and skincare line. I wanted to do something different at my age, since I felt I truly had something special to offer. All the discipline and knowledge I had gained over the years could be put to good use, and I felt there was no reason why I couldn't develop my own line. Using a good quality product does help maintain your skin, and I wanted people to know they could look younger if they were to do certain things.

I wanted to popularize the roll-on serum I had developed, and the agencies were not fond of my using my actual age to do so. Not that they cared what I had to say about any kind of serum. They just didn't like my telling people I was older than perhaps they'd thought I was. I may have even lost a job or two over that.

So I did talk to my good friend Suzanne, about this quite a bit. "I don't know," I told her, "Maybe this is not the right thing to do. How can I be sure? And they might just think that . . ."

"Irene, stop that," she said. "Just look in the mirror. That's all you have to do. You don't have to prove anything. Take a look at everything you've done in your life."

To her, my face was my validation. And what she told me was what I needed to hear. I decided to go ahead, pursuing products that were good and effective, while using a conscientious approach. The product had been in development for some time by then, but we actually started selling it, exclusively through Amazon, on my seventieth birthday.

CHAPTER 3

Skincare
(Habits and Breakthroughs)

W hen Suzanne told me not so long ago that seeing my face in the mirror was all the validation I need to freely reveal my age, regardless of what some modeling agency reps may have thought about it, it made me think back to the time in my life when looking in the mirror horrified me. Many years ago, I had an auto accident, a terrible accident that came at the height of my career. It devastated me.

From so many angles, I was shattered—emotionally, mentally, and physically. I incurred a blowout fracture—my eye fell back and dropped down. It was very difficult for the doctors to repair. Back then, they didn't have the techniques and level of medical technology that is now available. And the injury was unique, so the necessary operation was not one they would typically perform.

It was a month before I realized it was not healing as I would have wanted it to. The skin on the left side of my face didn't match the skin on the right. And the scarring was unsettling. I would not use the word *disfigured* because I think that would be too severe, but my facial skin was highly damaged. I pursued several doctors to advise me and consult on how I might take care of this condition and repair the damage. Most would not even consider touching me. They told me, "We cannot do the surgery, or even reconstructive surgery, because you will not be happy with the results."

They didn't want to take the risk. To make things worse, the injured eye was the one that had been my "good" eye. I was born with a weak eye. I was supposed to wear a patch as a child, but of course, I did not, and that eye remained weak. Now I had only one eye to see out of well, and that was the one that was injured. They just weren't willing to do further operations and risk the sight in that eye. In my usual manner, I refused to be defeated and so I started exploring and searching for a doctor who would try to help me. And I found a doctor in Austin, Texas, who told me about a cutting-edge doctor on Fifth Avenue in New York, who wasn't a surgeon, but a scientist who was curing people with scars like mine using silicone.

I knew nothing about silicone. I believe this doctor was truly ahead of his time. He would apply these teeny droplets of silicone over time to repair skin. I called him immediately and asked if he would see me.

Dr. Norman Orentreich, widely regarded as the father of dermatologic cosmetic surgery, agreed to see me, and when I went to him, he told me, "I can help you."

I was elated. "Oh my God, this is wonderful news. How long will it take, Doctor?"

"Ten years."

I looked at him like he had two heads. "Ten years! Are you crazy?" This was during my time of life when I had been modeling, being photographed, socializing with celebrities and politicians, and all of it was important to me. "What do you do that could take ten years?" I asked.

"Well, what I do is take these tiny droplets of silicone and inject them. But it has to be done only a little at a time."

People weren't doing this at that time. Silicone use for medical procedures was unheard of. He was pretty much the only doctor doing it. A lot of patients would not do it because they could not know what the results would be. I said, "Go for it. I'm your guinea pig. I want to do it."

I would go and see him three or four times a year, and in the beginning, up to five times. He would apply these droplets of silicone, and I didn't see much difference, but I wasn't giving up. The next year and the next, I kept at it without much change, but then I started seeing tiny improvements where my skin was no longer puckered down. When you have scars, that is where your skin folds in, but now it was starting to lift. It was very encouraging. This did, indeed, go on for ten years. As time went by, I would go in for maintenance. By then, his roll call was high with celebrities, politicians, and other doctors. He had come to be quite high up the ladder.

Well, here I am at seventy-five, rather than twenty. My face is much better in terms of the accident scarring. Believe it or not, I find myself contemplating having a mid-facelift. Some doctors did suggest it, and I thought, *Okay, this probably will make me look better.* Though, since I was writing this book, I hesitated. So I went to my husband and Suzanne to talk it over. She said, "Don't be ridiculous. Many women get surgery and still write books." Cosmetic surgery would not disqualify me from writing a book and talking about natural breakthroughs, as I had been contemplating.

Well, for now, I've put the idea of getting surgery on the back burner. Before anyone steps into having surgery, there are so many things to do and think about first. A little bit of something done to your face can go a long way. Micro drops are key, I think. Those silicone drops made a tremendous difference for me—the treatment brought about the changes slowly, but it actually worked. Taking the plunge into surgery is the last resort.

Healthy Habits for Glowing Skin

What really makes your skin glow? Many people spend a fortune trying to get that kind of great skin, or rather sustain it. Yet, you may be surprised to learn that the five habits of people with truly great skin are common habits that can change your skincare game for good. What if I told you, all you need are their simple secrets that you, too, can easily put to good use?

They cleanse. Don't mind the light bulbs and exclamation marks that pop in your head as you go through each habit. Yes, cleansing daily is one of the top five habits of people with great skin, and surely you can understand why. Your skin goes through the day with exposure to all sorts of things. The pores get clogged as a result of dust, dirt, and oil in your makeup, leaving you at risk of breakouts. Washing your face and skin at least twice daily, including once before bed, can clear impurities and keep your skin refreshed.

They protect their skin from the sun. And by this protection, I mean the proper, regular use of sunscreen. A good sunscreen will defend your skin from harmful UV rays, thus helping to prevent premature skin aging, pigmentation, and fine lines.

They take exercising seriously. Exercising is a thing, and a vital one, to be done regularly for your physical and skin health. People with great skin find the time to exercise and sweat out impurities. The skin glows naturally after a healthy exercise session, due in part to increased blood circulation giving the skin an extra boost of oxygen.

They ditch the unhealthy habits. There are some habits that spell doom for your skin, and top of the list is smoking. Check this out yourself: People with great skin are not chronic smokers or drinkers. Smoking accelerates wrinkles and dulls the skin, as well as staining your teeth and gums.

They eat healthy. The importance of healthy meals to skin health cannot be mentioned enough. Less oily foods and snacks as well as veggies and fruits can make a remarkable difference in your skin health. Focus on eating antioxidant-rich foods, fruits, and veggies. Plus, hydration is a must. *Drink water regularly.*

So there you have it, plain and simple. The thing about a habit is, it needs to be a consistent part of you. That's the only way to cash in on these habits for your skin's benefit.

Six Dermatological Breakthroughs to Defy Age

While we may not yet be able to bathe in the Fountain of Youth, science is getting much closer to keeping us ageless . . . at least, when it comes to our skin. Advancements in dermatological care have produced remarkable results for those seeking to defy age a little longer without going under the knife. Here I present what I believe to be the six most significant breakthroughs of recent years:

- **Fractional CO2 Laser Skin Resurfacing**
- **Vitamin A**
- **Helioplex and Mexoryl SX**
- **Advanced Wrinkle-Filling Injections**
- **Antioxidants**
- **Peptides**

Fractional CO2 Laser Skin Resurfacing: This procedure has a drastically shorter recovery time compared to earlier types of laser treatments or deep chemical peels. The fractional CO2 laser essentially bores out "columns" of skin, leaving healthy tissue untouched around them to aid in the healing process. After healing is complete, patients see a significant reduction in discoloration and wrinkles. The new skin cells that emerge are free of sun damage and contain more collagen than those they have replaced. Overall, skin has a more even tone and greater firmness.

The process is quick, but not entirely painless. An invasive treatment, the resurfacing requires numbing creams, and usually, injections of local anesthetics. It is not uncommon for pain medication to be prescribed afterward. Immediately following the procedure, the skin feels as though it has been badly sunburned and tightens so as to make facial expressions and even speaking uncomfortable. Side and stomach sleepers must also take care to sleep on their backs so that the copious amounts of moisturizer they are required to wear at night does not rub off on bed linens, leaving their skin unprotected.

Once dead skin begins to slough off, the face will be itchy and irritated. New pink skin will reveal itself under the flaking skin, and this pinkness can take several additional days to fade. During the entire recovery time—especially during the first three to four days—sunlight should be completely avoided. For deep scarring or serious discoloration, multiple treatments may be required. At nearly $5000 per treatment, this procedure is best for those willing to take sufficient time off for full recovery. But it does yield some of the most drastic effects, and it is thought to last for several years.

Vitamin A: Those who want to forego laser treatment for the time being still have many options when it comes to taking advantage of dermatological science to achieve younger looking skin. A University of Michigan study published in 2007 showed that over-the-counter retinol (ingredients chemically related to vitamin A) could improve skin firmness when applied three times weekly over a period of twenty-four weeks. Retinol and its prescription-strength counterparts, retinoids, are believed to inhibit collagen breakdown in cells of mature skin. Additionally, they may increase and regulate collagen production. This means firmer skin for you.

Before starting a patient on a prescription retinoid regimen with Retin-A or Renova, many dermatologists will suggest first using retinol products for a period of time so that the skin can adjust to the mild irritation that sometimes manifests in the form of dryness and redness. While it would be a misnomer to say that retinol and retinoids lead to photosensitivity of the skin, it is true that the vitamin A compounds themselves break down in the presence of sunlight. For this reason, you tend to see these ingredients used in night creams, where they will be most effective.

Helioplex and Mexoryl SX: Created by Neutrogena and L'Oréal, respectively, these two ingredients have changed the game of anti-aging sunscreens.

While producers of sunscreens containing the active ingredients *avobenzone* and *oxybenzone* have made the claim that they protect against both UVA and UVB rays, protection from UVA rays is, in fact, limited because these ingredients break down in sunlight. Essentially, after a period of sun exposure, the UVA protection factor in many sunscreens has disintegrated, allowing long UVA rays to penetrate to deeper layers of the skin and break down collagen and elastin. In addition, UVA rays are now known to contribute to the development of skin cancer.

Helioplex and Mexoryl SX stabilize these ingredients so that they resist breaking down, thus increasing the effectiveness of anti-aging sunscreens and reducing exposure to cancer-causing rays.

Advanced Wrinkle-Filling Injections: Dependent on our natural skin cycle, creams and serums generally require several weeks of continuous use before significant results are noticeable. Wrinkle injections, however, provide instant results by adding volume to skin exactly and only where desired. They are also much more natural looking and far less painful than surgery, with side effects generally limited to mild, temporary swelling or irritation at the injection site.

Botox, Perlane, Juvéderm, and Radiesse have emerged onto the market and generated great excitement among customers. Those who have enjoyed the effects of the widely popular filler, Restalyn, may benefit most from Perlane, a "thicker" version of the filler. Juvéderm has gained notoriety because not only does it act as an effective filler, but it even contains hyaluronic acid, which has been shown to generate collagen production and disrupt its breakdown.

The price of injections usually ranges from $500 to $1000 per syringe, and results last about a year or longer, making this a great option for those unafraid of needles and with money to spend.

Antioxidants: Consuming a diet rich in antioxidants is recommended for good health. We now know that topically applied antioxidants are also effective for protecting skin from the damaging free radicals with which we're constantly bombarded through exposure to air pollution or sunrays. Essentially, these free radicals are unstable molecules that "steal" electrons from the structures that make up a healthy skin cell. This impairs the cell's functions and slows down regeneration. Antioxidants are highly attractive to these free radicals, essentially intercepting them before they damage our cells.

While products containing antioxidants CoQ10 and vitamins C and E have been on the market for a while, discovery of the *coffee berry* has been particularly exciting to researchers. Often found near the equator, this fruit thrives in conditions of intense sun exposure. Many studies have found that the potency of antioxidants from this fruit is much greater than that of other antioxidants, which means greater protection for us. The best-performing *cosmeceuticals* (a term the cosmetic industry uses to refer to cosmetic products that have medicinal or drug-like benefits) seem to combine several complementary antioxidants for extra protection.

Peptides: For biologists, *peptide* is a nonspecific word that refers to the amino-acid chains that make up protein.

In cosmetics, the word *peptides* refers to a select few of these amino-acid chains. Palmitoyl pentapeptide-3, known commercially as *Matrixyl*, is one such peptide. It has been shown to stimulate collagen production in the skin. Collagen gives our skin firmness, but it breaks down over time. As we age, our skin loses the ability to recognize when collagen needs to be replaced. Matrixyl signals our cells to restart collagen production, thus firming our skin over time.

While Matrixyl is the most widely used peptide in skincare, there are others that work to boost collagen production or to address other skin concerns. *Argireline*, for instance, is a wrinkle-relaxing peptide that affects the face in a manner similar to that of Botox. This peptide blocks neurotransmitters that signal muscle contraction—but without the toxicity of the Botox agent. As research on Argireline continues, we can hope that an even better delivery system will increase efficacy of the peptide and provide a safer, equally effective substitute for Botox.

Ultimately, we must individually consider the cost, time, and relative benefits of each skincare treatment or regimen before determining what is best for ourselves. I have seen friends experience great results with fractional CO2 laser skin resurfacing, while others opt for new, advanced topical creams, not being able to accommodate the downtime associated with a laser procedure. In the end, a trusted, board-certified dermatologist can be a valuable liaison to the world of skincare science.

Healthy Habits for Overall Health

Every morning, I get up and put half of a lemon in a cup of hot water. Drinking this cleans your system, opening it up to receive your food and whatever else you decide to drink. It is good for you and your entire system. At night, before going to sleep, I take a bath in Epsom salt, which is so good for your joints and helps you relax. Between the two routines, lemon in hot water in the morning and Epsom salts at night, these are very healthy things to do.

During the day, of course, there are other types of conditioning and regimens and disciplines it would be wise to make routine. And don't forget to exercise. No athlete builds their skill by working out once a week. Exercise takes repetition and dedication along the lines of a daily routine, just as you would need in caring for your face to achieve desired results.

I do yoga three times a week and lift weights a couple of times a week. And I ride horses. I am an avid equestrian, and have ridden all over the world. So I must maintain my body. It is just a good idea to have healthy habits.

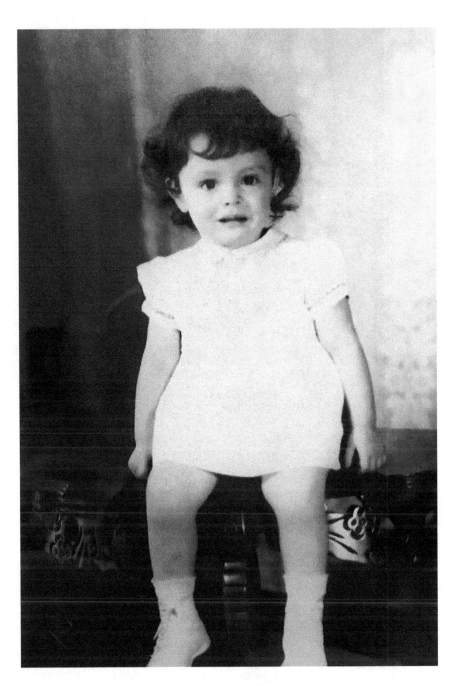

Early Childhood – Age 4

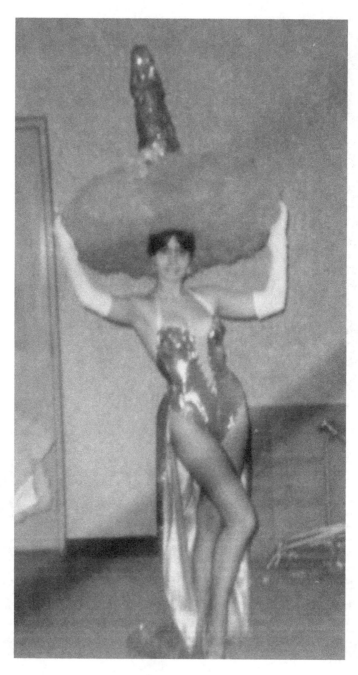

Dancing my way to Broadway

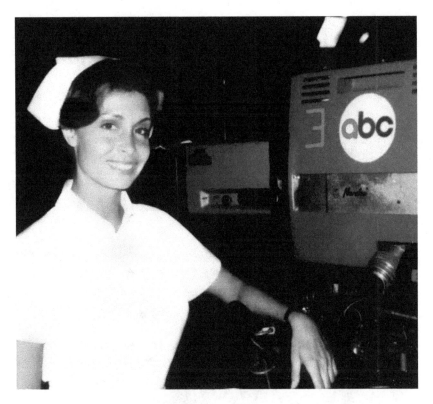

Landed a recurring role on the popular soap opera, General Hospital

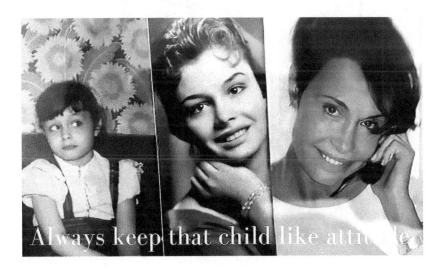

Always keep that child like attitude

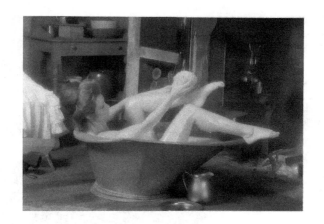

Early Modeling Shot

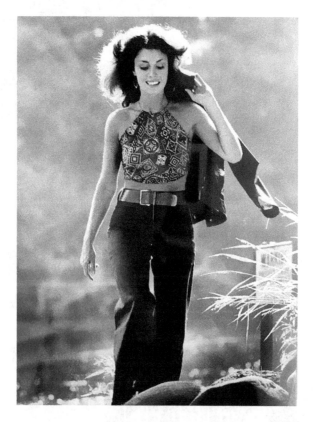

Early Modeling Shot

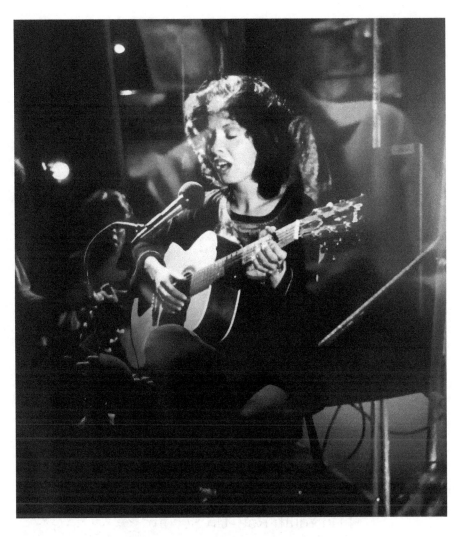

Early performance, playing guitar at "Ratso's" in Chicago...
a jazz club on Lincoln, north of Fullerton.

Life&Style

MIRACLE IN A BOTTLE

ROLL-ON RADIANCE!

To deeply moisturize and soften fine lines, this clever antiager holds up to 300 times its weight in water on your skin. Just as exciting? Its unique delivery system : a stainless-steel roller-ball that cools the skin while amping cellular turnover.

I On Youth Roll-On Serum by Irene Michaels, 43$, amazon.com

Life & Style Weekly Magazine deems I On Youth Collection by Irene Michaels™ Roll-On Serum a "Miracle in a Bottle" February 2016 Buy yours here: https://www.amazon.com/gp/product/B00Y4C6ZP4

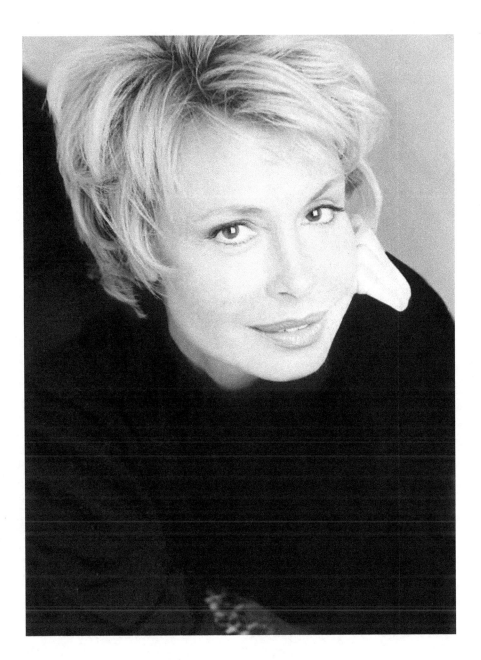

As a Blonde

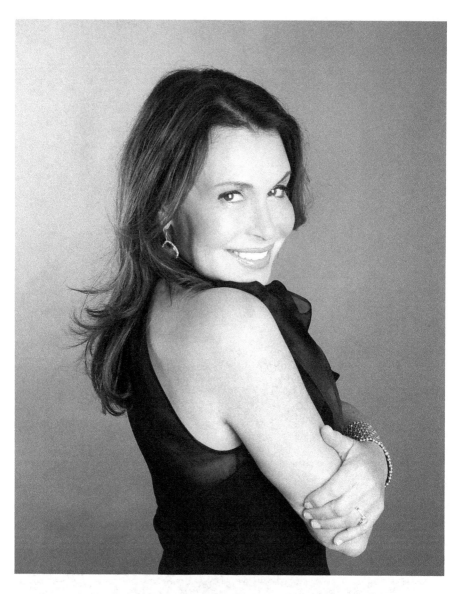

Later modeling shot Photo credit: Lisa Gottschalk

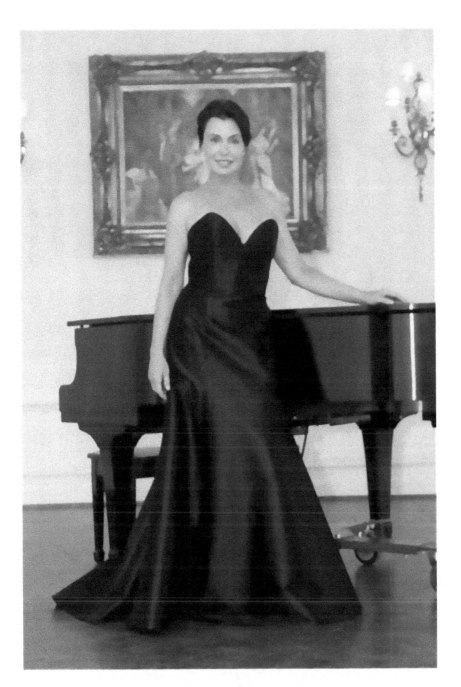

Later modeling shot

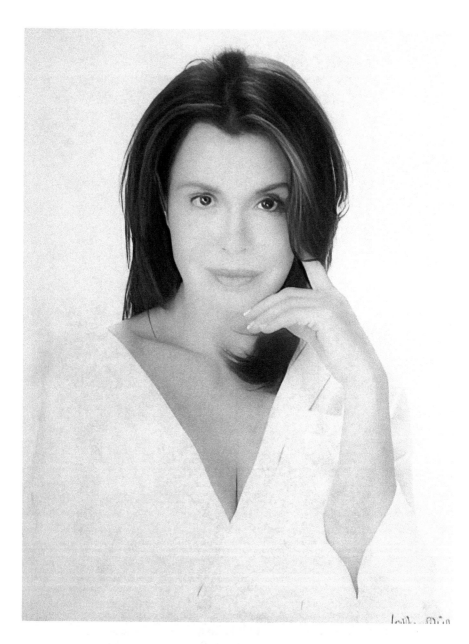

Later modeling shot

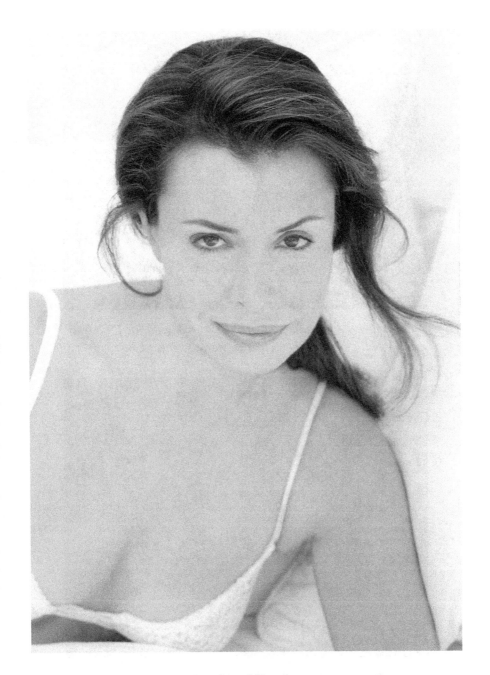

Later modeling shot

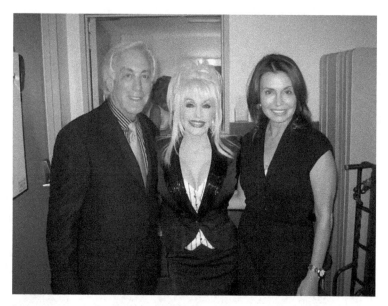

Pictured with Arny and Dolly Parton backstage at the Broadway
Opening of the musical 9 to 5 at The Marquis Theatre April 30, 2009

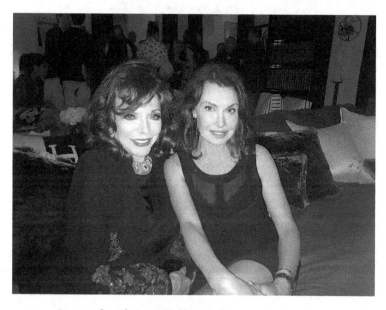

Pictured with Joan Collins OBE at a private party
celebrating the 75th Golden Globe Awards, January 6, 2018

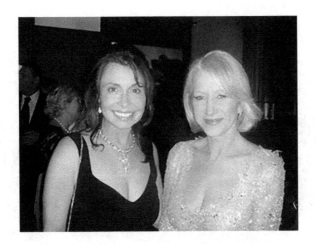

*Pictured with Dame Helen Mirren at the 2017
Chicago International Film Festival Spring Gala*

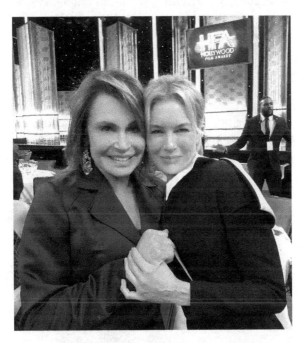

*Pictured with Renee Zellweger at the 23rd Hollywood Film
Awards which were held on November 3, 2019. That night
Renee received the first of 8 awards for her role as Judy Garland
in the biopic Judy, a film about Judy Garland's chaotic life.*

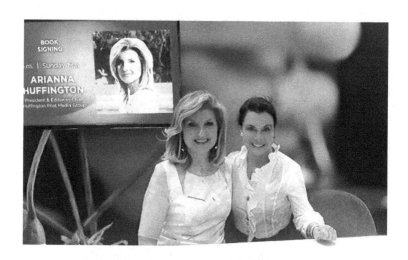

Thrive book signing with Arianna Huffington in Chicago on May 17, 2015. Contributing to the Huffington Post while Arianna was at the helm was great!!! My articles appeared in multiple sections and some are used in I On Beauty

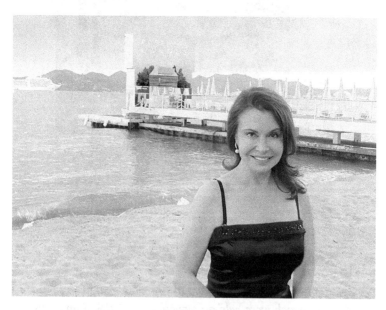

The 69th Cannes Film Festival which was held May 11 to 22, 2016 and I On The Scene was there.

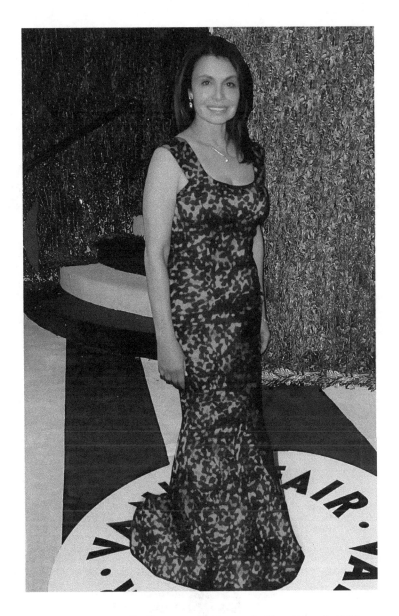

Vanity Fair's 2015 Oscar® party which was held in Beverly Hills, at a custom-designed space that connected the Wallis Annenberg Center for the Performing Arts with City Hall. On Oscar evening, February 22nd, guests entered through the Annenberg Center and I On The Scene was there.

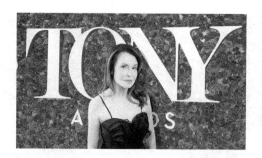

Arny was one of the producers of The Band's Visit which won 10 TONY AWARDS, including BEST MUSICAL, at the 72nd Annual Tony Awards on June 10, 2018 and I On The Scene was there.

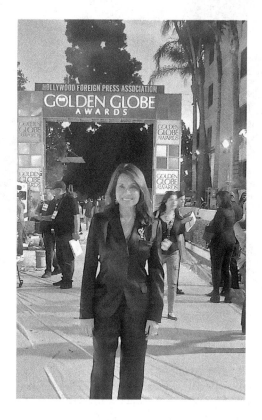

The 70th Golden Globe Awards honoring the best in film and television of 2012, was broadcast live from the Beverly Hilton Hotel in Beverly Hills, California on January 13, 2013, by NBC and I On The Scene was there.

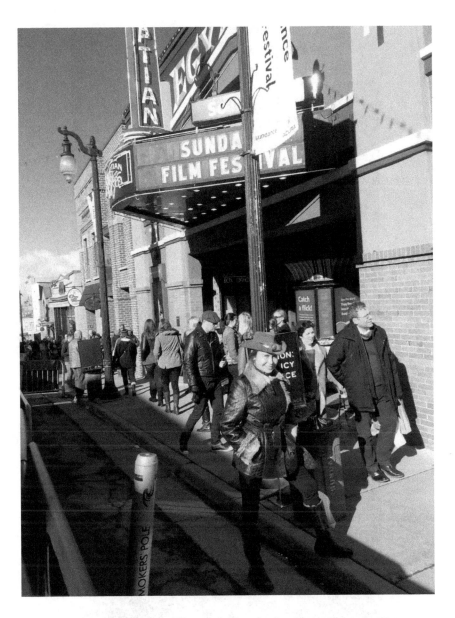

The 2015 Sundance Film Festival took place from January 22 to February 1, 2015. What Happened, Miss Simone?, a biographical documentary film about American singer Nina Simone, opened the festival. Comedy-drama film Grandma, *directed by Paul Weitz, served as the closing night film and I On The Scene was there.*

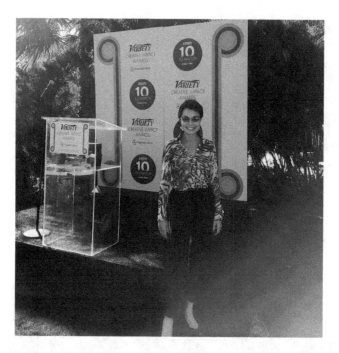

Mercedes-Benz marked the tenth anniversary of its collaboration with Hollywood's top actors and actresses in 2014 at the 25th Annual Palm Springs International Film Festival and I On The Scene was there.

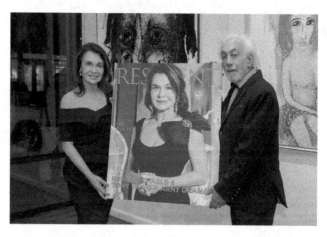

Irene and Arny, hosted an intimate evening at George Berges Gallery in SoHo to celebrate their Resident *cover on March 12, 2019. Photo credit: Suzanne Tripaldi*

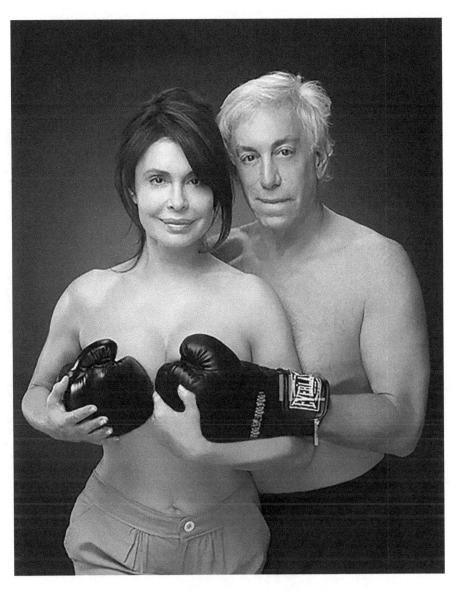

IRENE MICHAELS & ARNY GRANAT: A KNOCK-OUT COUPLE
Resident Magazine January 9, 2019 Photo credit: John Reilly

CHAPTER 4

Hyaluronic Acid
(Your Next Skincare Favorite)

This book is all about inspiration, and that's what I want to do by sharing my secrets. I am always asked to share my secrets with other women because I have so many to share. Not so surprising as I have worked the red carpet quite a bit, and I have had discussions with many celebrities who have shared theirs with me over the years.

Everyone would probably like to roll back the clock and get rid of that dry skin or those fine lines. I was on a quest to get rid of wrinkles, or at least minimize them. There are so many cosmetics out there that just don't work. So I set out on developing my own product line, which I finally did—I On Youth Collection by Irene Michaels™.

The Roll-On Serum uses a stainless steel rollerball for application, and is cool on the skin. You apply it under the eye in the morning and in the evening. It hydrates at a very deep level, nourishing the cells and energizing the skin's natural renewal process. The serum is an advanced skincare formula that rejuvenates your skin.

Now, is it permanent? I would not say that, but you certainly will get significant benefits since it holds in the moisture so well. The roll-on serum contains *hyaluronic acid*, a natural moisture magnet, and that is what we need to plump up the skin. The specialized molecules of hyaluronic acid retain up to 300 times their weight in water in your skin, diminishing wrinkles. Dull skin is revitalized since the serum promotes rapid cellular regeneration. These new, undamaged skin cells provide a flawless-looking skin for a radiant, refreshed appearance.

Now it can be used on more than just the face. You can target problem areas using the unique stainless steel roller ball, which is hypoallergenic and cool to the touch. It offers a smooth and precise application, not only around the eyes, but also along the lip line and creases of the nose, or even between the bust line and on the hands. Men will find it beneficial to use as well.

This serum is paraben-free and nontoxic, a wholesome product that is also cruelty-free, never having been tested on animals. I invested much research and effort in developing a product I could be proud to put my name on, and that is exactly what I did.

I On Youth Collection by Irene Michaels™ Roll-On Serum

- Roll back the clock on fine lines and dry skin
- A natural moisture magnet—hyaluronic acid
- Revitalize dull skin through rapid cellular regeneration
- Target problem areas using a unique roller ball for precise application
- Paraben-free, nontoxic, and cruelty-free (never tested on animals)

(Available for purchase exclusively on Amazon at: https://www.amazon.com/gp/product/B00Y4C6ZP4)

Benefits of Hyaluronic Acid

Women (and yes, men as well) try managing their skin in the best way possible so that it stays in great condition. And it is not surprising. Great skin gives you a great appearance overall, and that makes you feel so good.

Hyaluronic acid offers a lot of benefits for the human body in a number of ways. In the context of skincare, its natural ingredients are a boon for moisturizing skin and fighting signs of aging. Let's get started by considering some benefits of hyaluronic acid that people concerned with giving their skin the best possible care should know about.

- Protects Skin from UVB Rays
- Enhances Production of Collagen
- Enhances Skin Layers
- Moisturizes Skin

Protects Skin from UVB Rays: UVB rays emitted from the sun are extremely dangerous for human skin. Whenever you step outside your home, you need to protect your skin from the damaging effects inflicted by these rays. Hyaluronic acid protects your skin from UVB rays and minimizes various risks like sunspots and suntans.

Enhances Production of Collagen: Hyaluronic acid is essential for the production of collagen, which is an important protein in the human body. Collagen is an immense support for the structure of the skin, helping to make wrinkles and other signs of aging disappear. It also hides the skin discolorations that can start emerging after a certain age.

Enhances Skin Layers: Hyaluronic acid greatly enhances the layers of human skin, repairing skin tissues and protecting them from various sources of damage. It also improves the skin layers by hydrating and moisturizing them. Plumping the skin through hydration using hyaluronic acid immediately improves the appearance of crepey skin.

Moisturizes Skin: Skincare is a prodigious topic these days. Everyone, it seems, is focused on keeping their skin young and beautiful. As we start to age, our skin loses its moisture. This loss is not only due to aging, but a lot of people happen to have an extremely dry skin type. But that does not mean you cannot make it right, or at least, make a real effort to moisturize it.

Hyaluronic acid aids in deeply moisturizing your skin. If your skin is not well hydrated, then it will lose its firmness, and the signs of aging will start appearing too soon. This acid is nothing less than magic—it moisturizes your skin perfectly. It provides all the necessary hydration to your skin, preventing it from displaying the signs of aging, even going so far as to make it appear young and beautiful and fresh. And in a time when you are likely using much more hand sanitizer than usual, which can have a drying effect on the skin, look for one that has hyaluronic acid as an ingredient. This is so beneficial in replenishing moisture—it is what I am using during the pandemic.

I On Youth Collection by Irene Michaels™ Roll-On Serum

I have enjoyed a career in the entertainment industry for decades. Being so often in front of the cameras, I have gleaned a lifetime's worth of beauty tips from stars, public figures, colleagues, and friends. I am often asked how I am able to maintain my looks so well at my age. Not only does this make me feel great—who doesn't love a compliment?— but it also gives me the chance to help others feel great. I love seeing women shine when they feel beautiful.

A solid skincare routine should be seen as an investment in yourself. Yet, it can be difficult to know where to begin. The truth is, when it comes to skincare, there aren't secrets. It's science, and in this information age, the research is available to you. The difficulty is in separating fact from fiction. Some products are overpriced and overhyped. We have all tried expensive products that promised miracles and didn't deliver the results we expected. Thankfully, that is where you can benefit from my experience. I have been experimenting with beauty products and all their various ingredients for more than thirty years.

We all have different skin concerns, but one of the most pervasive is the need to treat fine lines and wrinkles. For people like me, a full night of beauty sleep just doesn't do it anymore! But even from your late twenties onwards, you can make a big difference in your appearance by treating this early sign of aging. By far, one of the best ingredients for this is hyaluronic acid. It has been a buzzword for a while now, and for good reason. Hyaluronic acid, despite its scary name, is a very gentle compound that occurs naturally in the body. It actually binds moisture to the collagen fibers in your skin to deeply moisturize and plump cells, leaving you with less-visible lines and wrinkles.

Exploring the beauty counters for a product with hyaluronic acid, I found many options, but I wasn't in love with any of them. I probably brought home over fifty samples of products, and over the course of a few months, crossed them off my list one by one. They were either too heavily scented (and naturally, you don't want anything competing with your signature fragrance) or didn't absorb well into the skin. Some had only a small amount of hyaluronic acid in them at all and left a strange, flaky residue. Others had impractical applicators. I saw an opportunity here. If I couldn't find what I wanted, I knew there would be other women in the same boat.

So I developed the I On Youth Collection by Irene Michaels™ Roll-On Serum. Containing hyaluronic acid, this deeply hydrating compound holds up to 300 times its weight in water on your skin, leaving your face richly moisturized for all-day comfort. The serum also nourishes tired skin, increasing the rate of cellular renewal to reveal a refreshed, more youthful complexion. And this roll-on serum can be used on more than just the face.

This serum includes another natural component found within the skin called *sodium PCA*, which helps protect skin from future damage by increasing its resiliency. And the addition of antioxidants such as vitamins C and E has the effect of reducing oxidative stress and damage to skin, and can stimulate new collagen growth.

Overall, this serum is exactly what was missing from the beauty counters and from my beauty routine. It has exactly what you need and doesn't have an inflated price to pay for all the things you don't. This new formula is paraben-free, which I believe is extremely relevant. Skincare should be wholesome, not toxic. In February 2016, *Life & Style Weekly* magazine called I On Youth Collection by Irene Michaels™ Roll-On Serum a "Miracle in a Bottle."

I am especially excited that the serum comes as a roll-on. The serum's stainless steel roller is cool to the touch and allows for precise application so that no serum is wasted. It is so much more convenient than a dropper or spray—especially when you're jet-setting all over the place.

It's All about Inspiration

"How do you look so good at your age?" Men and women ask me that question on almost a daily basis. Of course, some of it is genetic, but truly to a great extent, I attribute it to using my serum. When I started using hyaluronic acid, I was very impressed with how my skin felt, and after a few applications, how my small wrinkles seem to lesson quite a bit. That was enough for me to believe in the product and to promote it to others.

I have been so pleased to have a product I could always rely on to make me appear close to flawless for an award show I was covering or a TV appearance. What I absolutely love about my serum and its design is how convenient it is to take out of your purse and apply near your eyes. Not only does it feel good, but it's easy to use. It travels so well and doesn't take up any room. Most women who have my product love the size of it, the ease of applying it, and the results they receive.

All of us, if we live long enough, will experience an array of incidents, good and bad. In living with some of the traumatic things that have happened to me concerning my appearance, I had to find something to make me look better and feel better. I never forgot that feeling, and it has inspired me to share what I've learned with other women. I have always been a believer in helping others. It's good karma. I'm not vain; matter of fact, I'm pretty spiritual and I am not selfish. And it works. So why not share?

CHAPTER 5

Food for Staying Young

"Don't forget to eat your veggies." It still rings in my ears today after so many years. My mother used to tell me that when I was a kid, and it is the best advice. Wives tales of the informed and intelligent mothers of yesterday have lived with us throughout our lives. Eating healthy should always remain a part of our daily regimen, just a normal activity.

Eating vegetables is certainly a good idea. They're filled with chlorophyll, and they're just plain health-building. You don't want to be eating a lot of fatty foods, but that does not mean you must resign yourself to boredom. There are so many ways to design and make and cook and bake vegetables.

Here's a little trick I do to get down as many veggies as I can. I combine broccoli, cauliflower, Brussels sprouts, pea pods, carrots, and baked potato, and then I steam all of them and crush them together until they're almost the texture of meat. It tastes good, and its texture gives you that sensation of eating meat. Worth a try. It works for me.

A few years back when wheatgrass was big, I was juicing all my food. Now wheatgrass is good for you, but for me, it had an aftereffect of making me smell. "Only your friends would tell you this, Irene. You don't smell so well today." Now those are good friends. And it was coming out of my pores and on my breath. Every time I would speak, an odor would follow. I don't do that any longer.

But one thing I am still fond of—something that is quite healthy and even fun to do—is dehydrating my food. You buy a bunch of zucchini and tomatoes and cucumbers, slice them thin, almost potato-chip thin, and put them in the dehydrator. You could even sprinkle them with something like pumpkin seeds. I do mine overnight, so they come out quite crispy. You can put them in containers and have them on-hand all day for snacks—healthy, tasty, non-fattening snacks. So that's a good practice.

Of course, you want to always put herbs into your diet. Ginger is very good for digestion. I happen to enjoy flaxseed and seaweed, so I eat a lot of that. I also eat a lot of nuts, including raw cashews. And, as I said, pumpkin seeds.

It is better to not eat too much at any one meal. I never do because I don't like the way it makes me feel. Eating five small meals a day is the better choice rather than two big meals. Not only is it easier on your digestive system, it is good for your metabolism. People who want to lose weight will tell you one of the things they learn at these weight-loss clinics is a recommendation that you eat five times a day.

And speaking of weight loss, I do want to comment on some of those diet foods like Nutrisystem, Weight Watchers, and Jenny Craig. Well, I have tried them all. And the thing is, if you stop and think about it, they last forever. Some are frozen, though a lot of the food comes in a box. After sitting in a box over time, the food just isn't live. You're not eating anything live, so eventually, you just might feel somewhat dead as well. These foods are conditioned to last and the nutrients are just not there. It can be like eating hay. Be careful about these kinds of quick weight-loss diets. There are no shortcuts. You need to do the right thing, and do it often. And I think you'll find your body will respond.

A good idea, too, is to detox a couple of times a month. Now that doesn't mean you just don't eat, or that you limit yourself to liquids. They have these delicious detox soups, and they're pretty good. It gets the junk out of your body. If you detox for too long or too often you can loss valuable nutrients along with the toxins, leaving your body depleted. For this reason, I wouldn't recommend doing a "full-on" cleanse more than two to four times a year. Afterward, I always feel lighter with a little boost in energy. It is good for your brain and your brain's "muscle memory." When you eat certain things, your brain remembers that experience, and it can be a good feeling. There is nothing like sitting down to a good meal. All of this doesn't mean you can never eat meat. I advise eating a good piece of meat once in a while.

We are what we eat. No truer words have ever been said. And every time you recall those words should be like a celebration. I know that might sound funny, but it really is important. There's an old saying, *love makes the world go round.* Well, it should say, *love and food make the world go round.* I think that happens to be true.

When I was a kid, we had a designated time to sit at the table for dinner. My father would get home from work and my brothers would be coming in from school or some other activity, and I would be out doing whatever I happened to be doing. But we all got to the dinner table to sit down and eat together as we talked about the day's events. There was never a TV on in the background. People would talk to one another. Now, well the art of conversation at times can seem lost. It pains me to see.

The "smartphones" that have become ubiquitous are pretty dumb from my way of thinking. They've made walking mummies out of some children. You don't see their eyes any longer, just the tops of their heads. A parent who can get hold of those phones from their children as well as teach them some good eating habits will help them reap rewards later in life.

Six of the Best Foods for an Anti-Aging Diet

Youth is one of the biggest blessings one can be bestowed with, and even though it's priceless, it is limited. Youth is, perhaps, the most thriving and energetic time of one's life, when everything seems to be at its peak. That's why one of the biggest fears for many women is aging, and with it comes a wish to postpone the process as much as possible. There are various products on the market that claim to reduce aging and promise younger-looking skin. However, the best way to prevent aging is the natural way.

There are dozens of foods around you that are enriched with qualities to prevent aging and reduce the signs of aging. Here are some of the best foods you can use to prevent the signs of aging:

1. **Strawberries**

   Eating this delicious fruit is an excellent way to stop your skin from aging. It is rich in vitamin C and can help reduce wrinkles and dryness in the skin. Try them with other fruits rich in vitamin C—whole or in the form of a salad—on a daily basis for younger looking skin.

2. **Tomatoes**

   The tomato is a widely used fruit that has multiple benefits, including those that promote anti-aging. Tomatoes (and watermelons) contain lycopene, which causes your skin to be smooth and wrinkle-free. It also prevents sunburns and protects against harsh UV rays, as well as diminishes sun spots and age spots. The vitamin C in tomatoes boosts collagen production, which makes the skin firm and healthy. Consume tomatoes on a daily basis in the form of salad, paste, juice, or whole.

3. Tofu

Tofu is an excellent anti-aging food as it helps in making the skin more firm. It contains flavones, which ensure less wrinkles and smoother skin. Tofu, along with similar foods like soy milk, is an excellent choice to consume to prevent the skin from aging.

4. Tuna

Tuna has a long list of health benefits, and anti-aging is one, too. Tuna, as well as sardines and salmon, is rich in omega-3, a key ingredient in keeping your skin young and fresh. Omega-3 also prevents skin cancer. Consume tuna twice a week to ensure a glowing and younger looking skin.

5. Coffee

Believe it or not, coffee is beneficial for your skin in terms of its anti-aging properties. The caffeine in coffee tightens your skin's pores and also prevents skin cancer. Drink a cup or two of coffee on a daily basis to protect your skin from cancer.

6. Green Tea

Green tea is not just good for a detox, but equally good for your skin. Green tea is enriched with antioxidants and helps in flushing out the toxins from your skin. It also prevents your skin from developing wrinkles by protecting it against the sun. Drink green tea twice a day for flawless skin.

Try incorporating some, or all, of these foods as part of your daily eating regimen to achieve younger-looking and more-radiant skin in a matter of days.

Age-Defying Foods for Radiant Health

Diet is a necessary component in both physical and mental health. It is what determines how physically and mentally fit you are for coping with the daily challenges of life. All of us want to feel (and look) young forever. While that may not be exactly possible, these age-defying foods will help you preserve energy levels and look younger.

Olive Oil: Almost four decades ago, a group of researchers from the Seven Countries Study (SCS) conducted the first major study of the effects of diet and lifestyle (along with other risk factors) on cardiovascular disease across cultures and countries. They concluded that the monounsaturated fats found in olive oils are extremely beneficial for individuals suffering from heart diseases and cancer. Today, it is widely known that olive oil is a rich source of powerful antioxidants and polyphenols that prevent age-related diseases and make you feel young and healthy.

Lemons: The vitamin C found in lemons is great for your skin. It promotes healing and nourishes the skin. When lemon juice is applied to the skin, it has a bleaching effect that reduces age spots, freckles, and wrinkles. It is also a wonderful alternative to skincare products such as cleansers and toners.

Blueberries: As small as they may be, blueberries are packed with antioxidants and nutrients that are essential for the skin. The little fruits are rich in flavonoids, anthocyanins, and vitamin C, all of which reduce the aging process of skin cells. Daily consumption of blueberries also boosts memory and prevents the skin from wrinkling. It is important to mention here that the darker the color of the blueberries, the more beneficial they are. This is because the highest concentration of antioxidants is found in the darkest-colored berries. My personal favorite . . . I love to add them to a yogurt shake or steel cut oatmeal.

Leafy Greens: This is fairly obvious: green vegetables are wonderful for your physical and mental health. The dark leafy greens such as kale and spinach contain lutein and zeaxanthin, two powerful antioxidants that counter the negative effects of ultraviolet rays (from the sun) on the skin. When you go out in the sun, the ultraviolet rays cause inflammation, epidermal DNA damage, suppression of T cell-mediated immunity, and oxidative stress. This increases the risk of skin cancer and promotes aging. A higher intake of green vegetables, particularly leafy ones, can reduce these adverse effects.

Avocado: A scrumptious fruit, well-known for its anti-aging properties. It is filled with fatty acids that are healthy for the skin. The vitamins, nutrients, and unsaturated fats in an avocado provide the skin with the nourishment it needs. An avocado a day will help you attain a natural glow to your skin, all while reducing the signs of aging.

Whole grains: Daily intake of whole grains such as oats, barley, wheat, brown rice, and quinoa lowers the chances of heart diseases and type-2 diabetes. These whole grains are rich in fiber and help regulate the digestive system as well. Whole grains are essential for any anti-aging diet because of their multiple health benefits.

Yogurt: In the 1970s, it was reported that Soviet Georgia had the highest number of centenarians per capita compared to every other country in the world. Studies pointed to yogurt as the reason behind so many long lives. While there is no evidence-based science to support specific anti-aging properties of yogurt, this food is rich in calcium. Calcium helps maintain strong bone health and improves gut health, preventing several age-related illnesses such as weak bones and intestinal diseases.

Dark Chocolate: High-quality, dark cocoa is rich in flavanols, a powerful antioxidant that reduces inflammation and improves blood circulation. It also promotes the skin's ability to retain moisture, making it less prone to wrinkles and other age-related skin deformations.

Herbs for Ageless Beauty Regimens

There is a lot of power in nature. Researchers have long recognized the pharmaceutical value of naturally occurring compounds. Many of the potent chemicals in today's medicines were not first created in a lab, but rather harnessed from plants. When it comes to skincare, many doctors and other experts agree that certain herbs offer effective anti-aging properties important to a beauty regimen. Among the most highly recognized are *ginseng, sage, oregano, and rosemary.*

Ginseng: The anti-aging properties of ginseng are probably the best publicized of all the herbs. For thousands of years, ginseng has been used to enhance health and wellness in a variety of ways. Millions trust ginseng supplements to aid in cognitive function. When applied topically to the skin, this herb has been shown to brighten the complexion and increase radiance by stimulating blood flow and supporting cellular turnover. Ginseng's antibacterial properties help soothe inflammation. Further, it is rich in antioxidants, adding protection against free radicals that can damage surface skin cells.

Sage: Noted for its skin conditioning and astringent properties, sage is found in many facial cleansers. It is effective at removing impurities from the surface of the skin while soothing skin and reducing inflammation. Sage oil has also been said to help regulate sebum production, which is particularly helpful to those with oily skin. Antioxidants in sage deliver nutrients to the cells as well as shield against the harmful effects of free radicals.

Oregano: This yummy herb is not only a delicious staple of Mediterranean food, but it is also good for your body and great for your skin. Packed with omega-3 fatty acids, vitamins, and antioxidants, oregano has long been said to support a healthy immune system and fight colds, but its uses don't stop there. Its oil can also be used to treat inflammatory skin conditions such as rosacea and psoriasis. Some have had success mixing oregano oil with olive oil and applying it directly to the face to smooth out lines and treat age spots.

Rosemary: An aromatic favorite, rosemary is found in many skincare products. It supports collagen production and helps skin maintain moisture, both of which stave off the formation (or deepening) of lines and wrinkles. Like the other herbs mentioned here, it also contains many antioxidants to protect against damage caused by free radicals. Aiding in circulation and cellular turnover, rosemary contributes to a younger-looking, more radiant complexion. This herb's invigorating fragrance makes it one of my personal favorites, especially in products where it replaces artificial fragrances that can be irritating.

As you can see, these four herbs have a lot to offer in terms of anti-aging health and skincare. As always, be sure to talk to your doctor before incorporating new supplements into your diet and remember to dilute these potent oils before applying directly to your skin.

Teas to Soothe Body and Mind—and Skin

Tea has been clinically proven the best beverage for bringing anti-aging benefits to all layers of skin. Tea has less caffeine than coffee, and the antioxidant properties keep the body and skin always hydrated and healthy. However, as tea relaxes and soothes body and mind, it also brings many benefits to reduce the aging appearance of the skin. There are many teas out there with properties that are especially effective at promoting the anti-aging process, reducing wrinkles from the eye area, mouth area, and forehead.

Green Tea: Green tea can heal the body and skin as well. It has particular antioxidant properties that contain vitamin C, which is great for skin tightening and improves the skin collagen. The high antioxidant properties help to nourish the skin and slow down the aging process. Green tea fights bacteria that can cause many skin problems. Also, it reduces the cholesterol level, protects against heart diseases, and prevents cancer.

Black Tea: Black tea is the most common tea that can be seen on everyone's breakfast table. The flavonoid properties of black tea help the skin by promoting and improving the skin's texture starting from the skin beneath. It prevents the emergence of dull and damaged cells and helps to fight against wrinkles by increasing cell turnover. Black tea also improves bone strength, promotes healthy skin, and regulates the immune system in an effective way.

Ginger Tea: Ginger has antioxidant properties. Hence, it acts as an antioxidant by helping to reduce the stress that often leads to premature aging and wrinkles of the skin. The tea helps to strengthen the immune system, lower blood pressure, and manages diabetes. Ginger inhibits the enzymes that break down the collagen and elastin that promote skin elasticity. You may drink lemon-honey tea or lemon-ginger tea to get the best benefit.

Oolong Tea: Oolong tea is the most potent beverage for promoting healthy skin. It helps to reduce skin inflammation and removes skin blemishes. Drinking Oolong tea consistently regulates the skin layer and tightens the skin. Moreover, it nourishes and moisturizes the skin, helping to reduce dryness of the skin which leads the anti-aging appearance. Oolong tea fights against the bacterial radicals and the fine lines of the skin's appearance.

White Tea: Last but not least, is white tea, which is basically known for having the highest level of antioxidants and nutrients. White tea has antioxidant properties that aid in reducing premature aging and free radicals. As it contains maximum nutrients, adding white tea to your everyday routine will help you to improve skin collagen.

White tea protects the skin from sunburn and also it helps to rejuvenate the skin of dead skin cells and wrinkles. It promotes healthy skin and hair, as well as overall health by reducing fat and cholesterol levels, preventing cancer, and protecting the heart.

The Choices You Make Every Day

Keeping up with the necessary discipline in my overall regimen has come naturally to me. As a dancer, right from the time I was a young girl, I've always been disciplined. These are the words, that I like to call the 3D's of MY life.

~ Determination
~ Dedication
~ Diligence

It is okay to have a little vanity about your looks. Perfectly okay. I think it's actually healthy. It comes down to a little bit of personality. Some people don't care how they look, but I don't see that as healthy.

Another thing to keep in mind is that we would have to do really bad things to our body for it to just lie down and die. I suppose there is a better way to phrase that, but I just want to point out that our bodies are the toughest machines ever built. Nothing compares. Think of how many little muscles and nerve connections it takes to blink your eyes. The average person blinks 15 to 20 times per minute. That's up to 1,200 times per hour and a whopping 28,800 times in a day!

Just to pick up a button off a countertop takes the fingers, nerves, muscles, brain signals, all these reactions running through your body. An amazing thing! As I get older, I definitely am getting more and more into thinking about these kinds of things. If we can just be more balanced with our minds to do good for ourselves, eat well, be dedicated to ourselves, love ourselves, then I think we will be okay.

Now just to be clear, I do crave junk food. My junk food favorite is pizza. I'll sneak off and have a slice. Or ice cream. And I love Snickers bars. So that is what I binge on when I do. I just try to not keep too much of that on hand. Though, I am the kind of person who can eat one potato chip and stop. I also love to drink coffee. There's been some controversy off and on over whether coffee is good for you. But coffee, as I pointed out above, has real anti-aging benefits. Even skincare products have coffee in them at times. How bad could it be?

Just don't forget: We are what we eat. Inflammation can be a real source of our body's not feeling as well as it could. And yet, we may not even be aware of how our diets are full of things that create inflammation. We have inflammation in our body naturally, and sometimes the foods we eat can aggravate that reaction. That is something you might want to do a little research on and get a better idea of what that is all about. It is something I am learning about today.

I see a nutritionist who has taught me many things, Sherry Belcher. She started me on protein shakes, and they're very good.

RECIPE FOR MORNING SHAKE

What you need:

- Protein powder - 1 scoop
- Nano greens - 1 scoop
- Banana – ½
- Pumpkin Seed Oil - 2 oz.
- Vanilla Soy Milk - ½ cup
- Ice - ½ cup

Procedure:

- Put all ingredients in a blender and blend til smooth.

CHAPTER 6

Straight from Your Kitchen

I'm quite fond of the idea that people should pamper themselves. It's true that can be hard to do racing around in the fast-paced world we live in these days. But if you manage to sneak in a few hours a day, or even every other day, you can give yourself a treat. Start by putting some cucumbers on your face or over your eyes. Or you could use an ice mask. This will take away puffiness and feel very nice.

You could take a bath in Epsom salts—they even come in soothing scents, for instance, lavender or chamomile. Sometimes while I'm in the bathtub, I'll shampoo my hair and use apple cider vinegar afterwards to close all the pores and give my hair a nice shine. It also is good for people who highlight their hair, and for split ends. Using vinegar on your hair may sound terrible, and yes, some think it smells terrible.

At an early age, I did a lot of hair modeling. I dyed my hair blonde, red, black—you name it, I did it. And my hair was falling out! A friend gave me a whole bunch of tips and an apple cider vinegar rinse was one of them. Well, I tried it, and I ended up passing along this tip to other friends. Some of them loved it, couldn't thank me enough. Others, not so much. But in my opinion, it works, and I recommend you try it. Another point to keep in mind is that when women lose hair, it is often at the temples, and that is often where they start going gray. Brushing some apple cider vinegar through that area will help as well. It's not a full remedy, but it will help.

How to Make a DIY Body Scrub

Skincare is important because every woman wants to flaunt bright and attractive skin. To achieve this, you must maintain a healthy skincare routine that nourishes and rejuvenates the skin. This is where a soothing body scrub comes in. Body scrubs exfoliate the skin and eliminate dead cells that cause dullness and block your pores. Regular exfoliation helps the skin to stay fresh and clean, and brightens the complexion.

You can get a body scrub from the beauty shop and enjoy marvelous results, but why spend the extra cash when there are easy, inexpensive DIY body scrubs to choose from? Contrary to what you might think, creating a homemade body scrub involves common ingredients like brown sugar, oatmeal, banana, and essential oils. Here are some wonderful DIY recipes along with descriptions of their impacts on the skin.

OATMEAL AND BROWN SUGAR BODY SCRUB

Oatmeal is used as a great substitute for coffee in skincare. It is gentle on sensitive skin and helpful to treat skin issues. Brown sugar is also a major player in the skincare industry. It is used in place of white sugar because of its soothing, nourishing, and hydrating power.

What you need:

- Brown sugar - ½ cup
- Olive oil - ¼ cup
- Oatmeal - ½ cup
- Essential oil - 2–3 drops

Procedure:

- Mix all ingredients together in a bowl. Cleanse your skin, and then rub in the paste using small circular motions. Make sure the skin is wet when you do this. Leave it on for a few minutes and then rinse. You may also need to bathe or cleanse thoroughly afterward.

BANANA BODY SCRUB

The creamy nature of this fruit combined with its skin lightening and oil control properties make it a common staple for body scrubs. Use this scrub on oily skin for amazing results.

What you need:

- Ripe banana - 1
- Brown sugar - 1 tablespoon
- Vanilla (optional) - 1 teaspoon

Procedure:

- Mix the ingredients together slightly, leaving a little coarseness. Rub on your skin while in the shower and allow it to sit for a few minutes. After this time, massage the body in circular motions before rinsing.

YOGURT BODY SCRUB

Yogurt is a natural skin cleanser and moisturizer. Like the banana scrub, this recipe smells like dessert and is highly effective for glowing skin.

What you need:

- Yogurt - 1 tablespoon
- Olive oil - ¼ cup
- Granulated white sugar - 3 tablespoons
- Honey - 1 teaspoon

Procedure:

- Mix all ingredients into a coarse paste and apply on clean skin. Massage in circular motions for up to ten minutes. Wash off with lukewarm water.

GREEN TEA AND SALT BODY SCRUB

As I discussed in chapter five, there are many benefits from green tea to health and skin. This scrub uses both green tea and salt, which is a great combination to get smooth, supple skin.

What you need:

- Epsom salts - 3 teaspoons
- Baking soda - 3 teaspoons
- Green tea leaves - 1 bag
- Jojoba oil or olive oil - 4 tablespoons

Procedure:

- First, mix the Epsom salts, baking soda, and green tea leaves together. When that is done, add the oil and apply the mixture on the skin in circular motions. Rinse off after a few minutes.

How to Make a DIY Face Masque

A good day in the spa means closing your eyes under the nourishing influence of a face masque. The only problem is you might be too busy for this luxurious adventure. There's no hard rule that says a face masque can only be made and applied in a spa. In fact, in a few seconds, some helpful recipes will reveal that you can use humble food items like yogurt, oatmeal, and honey to create an effective DIY face masque.

A VINEGAR FACIAL AT HOME

Vinegar has proven to be one of the most important items in a home. It is useful in cooking, cleaning, and now, facials. Mix ¼ cup of water and a ¼ cup of apple cider vinegar. Apply on a clean face and leave to dry. It helps to tighten the skin and promote freshness.

OATMEAL MASQUE
TO FIGHT REDNESS

When you have been overexposed to the sun and can't get rid of the redness, look to a soothing and exfoliating oatmeal masque. This facial treats skin inflammation and also kills bacteria.

What you need:

- Oatmeal - 2 tablespoons
- Ripe Banana - ½
- Honey - 1 teaspoon

Procedure:

- Mash up the ripe banana and mix it with the other ingredients. Rub gently on the face for a few minutes, and then rinse off.

ALL-PURPOSE MILK FACE MASQUE

Some people search for a homemade masque that can treat specific skin problems. When you are unsure, you can use this milk face masque to get results and enjoy a fancy treat.

What you need:

- Powdered milk - ½ cup
- Water - enough to make a paste

Procedure:

- Make a thick paste by mixing the ingredients. Slather it on your face and allow it to dry completely. Rinse the masque off afterward with warm water.

MILK AND HONEY COMBO FACIAL

This face masque fights blemishes and treats acne-prone skin. It is a gentle, exfoliating masque. You would also benefit from the antibacterial property of honey for clean skin.

What you need:

- Honey - 2 tablespoons
- Nutmeg - 2 tablespoons
- Milk - 2 teaspoons

Procedure:

- Mix these ingredients together in a bowl, and then apply the mixture on the face. Allow the masque to sit for about fifteen minutes before rinsing with water. Don't forget to apply a soothing moisturizer afterward.

PUMPKIN SMOOTHIE MASQUE

Get that extra healthy glow with this smoothie masque. This smoothie is packed with beauty vitamins and nutrients. It is wonderful for the skin and body.

What you need:

- Canned pumpkin - ½ cup
- Frozen banana - ½
- Cinnamon - 1 teaspoon
- Almond milk - 1 cup
- Honey

Procedure:

- Blend all ingredients for one minute in a blender. Apply the smoothie on the face as a masque and enjoy the rest as a nourishing drink. Wait for a few minutes, then remove the masque with a damp washcloth. Rub in a moisturizing serum or cream afterward.

JUST PLAIN MAYONNAISE

For a clean and smooth face, plain mayonnaise from your refrigerator is all you need. Coat your entire face in mayonnaise and leave it to sit for twenty minutes. Wipe with a damp cloth and rinse with clean, cool water. This is great for all skin types.

DIY Masques to Make Your Hair Fabulous

A woman's mane is her pride, and most of us do not hesitate to spend hundreds of dollars at the salon trying to make it glow. Going to the salon is great for your hair and lets the professionals do their job. But most of the products and styling methods used in the salon actually can increase stress and damage to your hair.

The solution is to indulge yourself in some basic hair pampering and a quality-control routine using DIY hair masque. Hair masques are invaluable because they are quick and easy to use with ingredients that come straight out of your kitchen. These natural ingredients are super effective and necessary to maintain healthy, lustrous, damage-free hair. Remember to use these hair masques regularly for best results.

EGG HAIR MASQUE

Eggs are indispensable in a list of natural items to groom healthy hair. They contain protein, amino acids, and vitamin D. These nutrients help to strengthen hair follicles, lock in moisture, and promote growth.

What you need:

- Egg yolk - 1
- Olive oil - 1 tablespoon
- Honey - ½ tablespoon
- Ripe avocado - ½ (optional, for hair softness)
- Whole fat yogurt - 2–3 tablespoons (optional, adds strength and shine to hair)

Procedure:

- Place egg yolk, olive oil, honey, etc., in a bowl and mix well. You can add 2 to 3 tablespoons of water to thin out the mixture. Be sure to use cool or lukewarm water so the egg doesn't cook in your hair.
- If you are using an avocado, mash/blend it nicely before adding.
- Massage the final mixture into clean, damp hair. Cover with a shower cap and leave it to sit for 30 to 60 minutes. Rinse out and wash the hair with a mild shampoo. You can condition lightly, too.

Banana Hair Masques

Banana hair masques are rich and greatly beneficial to damaged or brittle hair. They help to prevent split ends, breakage, and hair aging. So, if you want to keep your strands youthful and thick, get started with a banana hair masque.

BANANA HAIR MASQUE #1

What you need:

- Ripe banana - 1
- Honey - 1 tablespoon
- Olive oil - 1 tablespoon

Procedure:

- Mash one ripe banana, or more depending on the volume of your hair. Add 1 tablespoon honey and 1 tablespoon olive oil. Blend the ingredients into a smooth paste and apply in small sections to clean, damp hair. Cover with a shower cap for 30 to 60 minutes, then shampoo and condition.

BANANA HAIR MASQUE #2

This hair masque is everything you ever wanted and can make your home feel like a spa.

What you need:

- Avocado - 1½
- Egg - 1 large
- Banana - 1½
- Olive oil - 1 tablespoon
- Apple cider vinegar - ¼ cup
- Water - 1 cup

Procedure:

- In a blender, add avocado, egg, banana, and olive oil. Blend into a smooth paste and massage gently into your hair. Leave it in for a few minutes and rinse out.
- Next, mix apple cider vinegar with water. Apply on the rinsed hair. Rinse out the vinegar water thoroughly after a few minutes.
- These ingredients work together to clean out dirt, prevent dandruff, and moisturize the hair and scalp. They promote healthy hair growth, leaving you with fuller, shinier hair.

COCONUT OIL AND HONEY HAIR MASQUE

If you have fine or medium hair, this hair masque is ideal to nourish your hair follicles and protect the natural hair proteins.

What you need:

- Coconut oil - 2–4 tablespoons
- Honey - 1 tablespoon

Procedure:

- Mix the coconut oil with the honey in a pot and heat it up so the honey and coconut oil melt into each other.
- Transfer the mixture into a bowl and let it cool.
- Add another tablespoon of coconut oil, if it's too thick. Wash your hair and apply the mixture in sections while the hair is damp. Cover with a shower cap for 30 minutes or more and rinse out.

AVOCADO, COCONUT MILK, AND HONEY HAIR MASQUE

Do you feel like your hair has lost its vibrant look? Try this recipe and enjoy soft, bouncy, vibrant hair.

What you need:

- Avocado - 1
- Unsweetened coconut milk - ½ cup
- Olive oil - 1 cup
- Honey - 1 tablespoon

Procedure:

- Combine avocado, coconut milk, and olive oil in a blender and slather on your hair. Tie the hair into a bun and leave the masque to sit this way for about one hour. Rinse and enjoy.

The Miracle of Mayonnaise

Fingernail strengthener: Do your fingernails break and seem weak? Or do you need them to stand out? Weak or ugly fingernails can put a dent in a beauty routine requiring perfectly manicured nails. Fret no more and dive into the miracle of mayonnaise. I mean this literally. Put a good amount of mayonnaise in a bowl and dip your fingernails in. Wash after 5 minutes.

Kill head lice: Head lice are nasty, and most times getting rid of them requires prescription medication. But not anymore, with mayo. For kids and adults alike, apply a good amount of mayonnaise on the scalp and hair before sleeping. Cover with a shower cap. Wash off with shampoo and use a fine-tooth comb to eliminate any remaining lice in the morning. Repeat this procedure for 7–10 days for permanent results.

Dry scalp relief: Dry, itchy scalp can be as good as gone with mayo on your beauty shelf. Apply a few tablespoons of mayo to your scalp and massage thoroughly with your fingers. Aside from helping to moisturize the scalp and eliminate the dryness and itch, the massage also promotes blood circulation.

Elbow and knee softener: Remember those stubborn patches of skin on the elbow and knee that always seem dry? Apply mayonnaise and rinse off after up to 15 minutes during a shower. The skin is moisturized, made supple and smooth.

And that is The Miracle of Mayonnaise!

Something Different

Along with all of these body scrubs and masques is another thing I think is good for you and kind of fun as well because you can put it on your body or you could simply eat it—coconut oil. Fresh coconut oil, right out of the bottle, anywhere on your body is so good, and if you scoop out a teaspoonful and eat it, it would be a very healthy thing to do.

While you are at it with pampering yourself, try lying down on the floor and putting your feet up on the wall. This is great to do every day for at least two minutes for your heart and your entire system. I've seen this help some women even look a little younger.

As we get older and watch our hair turn gray, it can be difficult. And this applies to more than just the hair on your head. Your hair, eyebrows, and pubic hair can all turn gray, and I don't want any hair on my body to be gray. There are spots on my body where I definitely will not be having anyone dye my hair. So one big trick and a tip for you to try is this: Take a teabag (or two or three) after it has been used and place that on your body over the pubic hairs and let it sit for about fifteen minutes. It will dye your hairs naturally. All I can say is that it works.

And speaking of hair, here's one more tip that I love: I don't always shampoo my hair with soap. There are these cleansing conditioners, and I brought one to my stylist. She said, "I don't want to use this. This doesn't make sense." I said, "Let's try it. We can always do something different next time."

Lo and behold, my hair looked so great, I've been using it ever since. My dear friend Suzanne had been the one to recommend that to me, and it was a great tip. It helps retain essential oils and to smooth the hair cuticles so they lay flat. My hair still looks pumped up and great the next day. However, you do need to use a shampoo after a chemical process.

Every autumn, Suzanne and I head for the Poconos to a destination spa we absolutely love—The French Manor Inn & Spa (https://thefrenchmanor.com 570-676-3244).

The sisters who own this combination spa retreat and inn, Genevieve Reese and Bridget Weber, know what it means to pamper their guests. The treatments, the food, the staff—all are wonderful and make our time there extraordinary. This stone chateau sits atop a mountain in a setting that is lovely and secluded. The rooms, the dining, and all accommodations are luxurious. We always look forward to our time there, and we are hopeful that we will be able to head there soon on our annual trip, this time to celebrate this book (in spite of COVID-19).

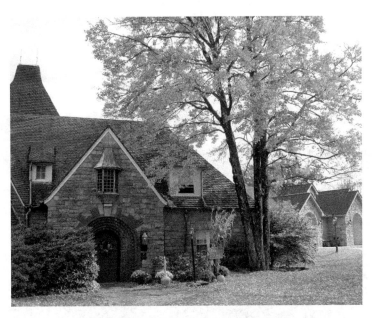

*Main Building of The French Manor Inn in the
foreground with the Spa Suites in the background*

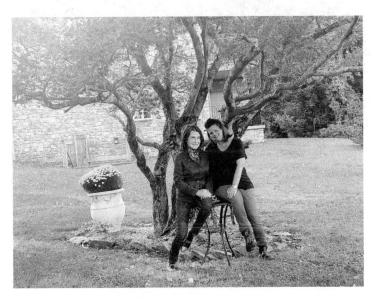

*Pictured with Suzanne on the grounds of
The French Manor Inn (October 9, 2020)*

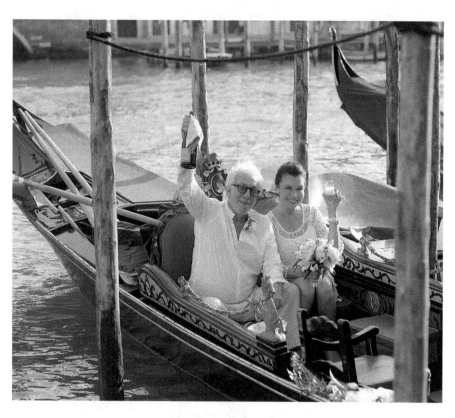

Venice Wedding July 2016

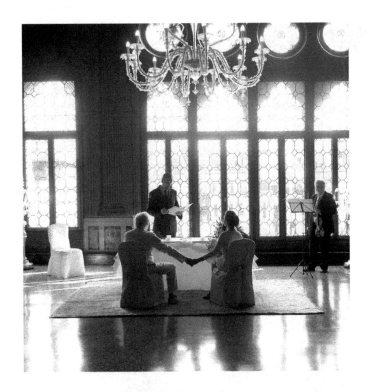

Venice Wedding July 2016

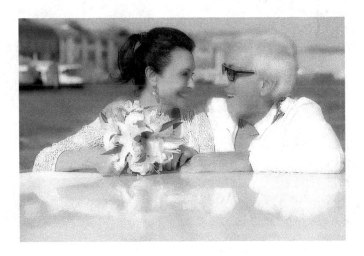

Venice Wedding July 2016

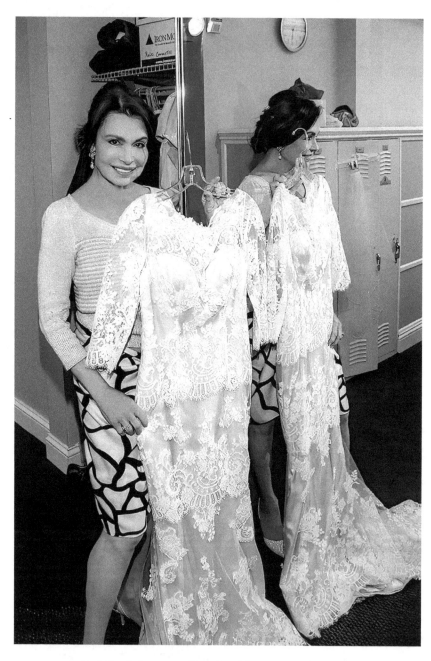

Oak Park Country Club Wedding November 2016
Photo Credit: Mitchell Canoff

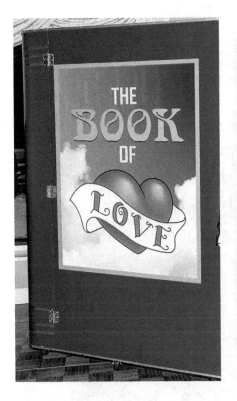

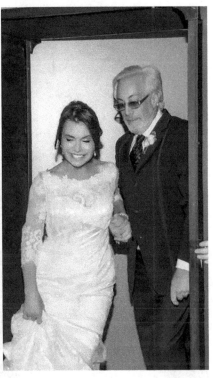

Oak Park Country Club Wedding
November 2016 Photo Credit:
Mitchell Canoff

Oak Park Country Club Wedding
November 2016 Photo Credit:
Mitchell Canoff

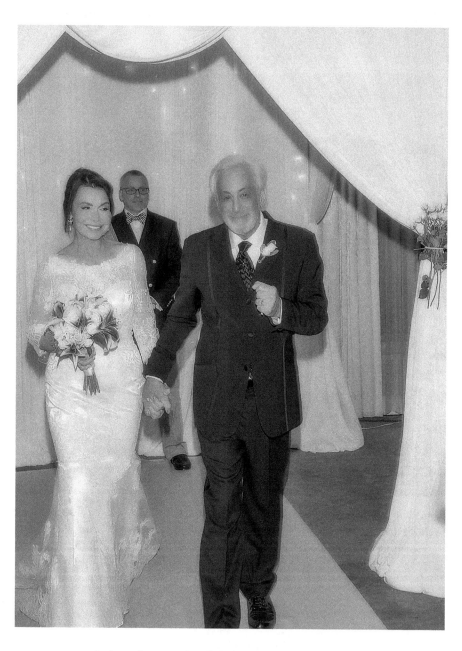

Oak Park Country Club Wedding November 2016
Photo Credit: Mitchell Canoff

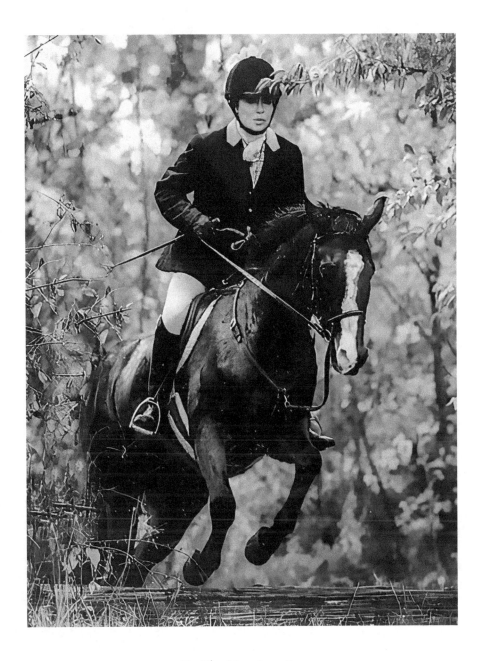

On The Marc in action

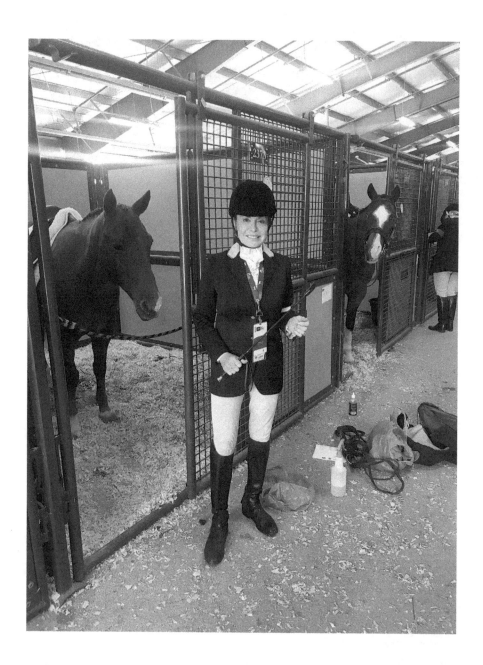

The Land Rover Kentucky Three Day Event is a sponsored competition that takes place in Lexington, Kentucky that year I served as an Outrider. The event took place April 25 – 28, 2019 and I On The Scene was there.

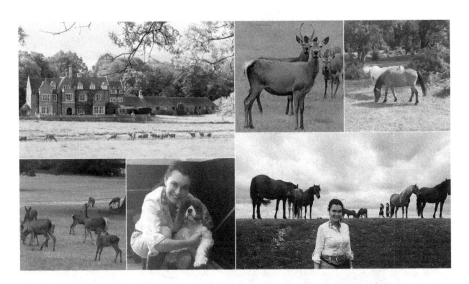

*Riding Weekend Burley Manor in New Forest National Park,
Hampshire England 2016 the nature images were taken
by yours truly, and I On The Scene was there.*

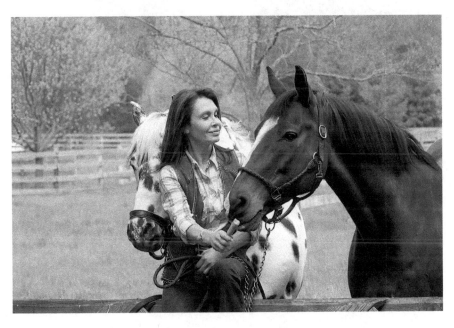

Spending time with Marc and Peek-A-Boo

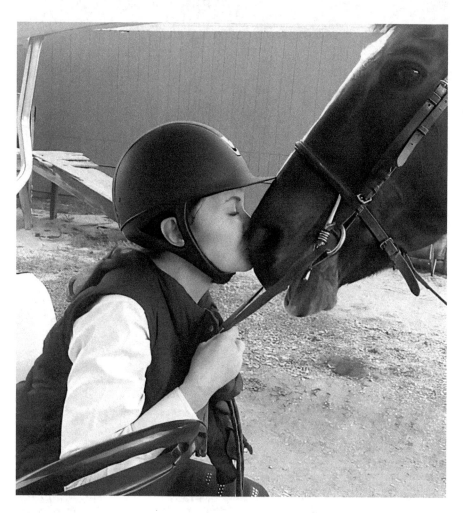

Just love this guy!

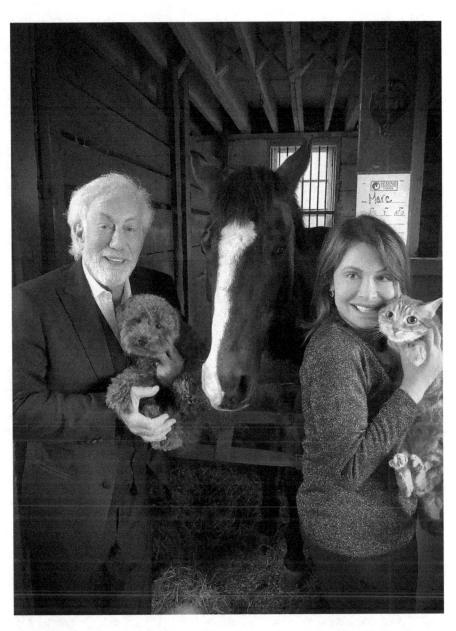

Our Holiday Photo with Rudy, Marc & Felix 2019

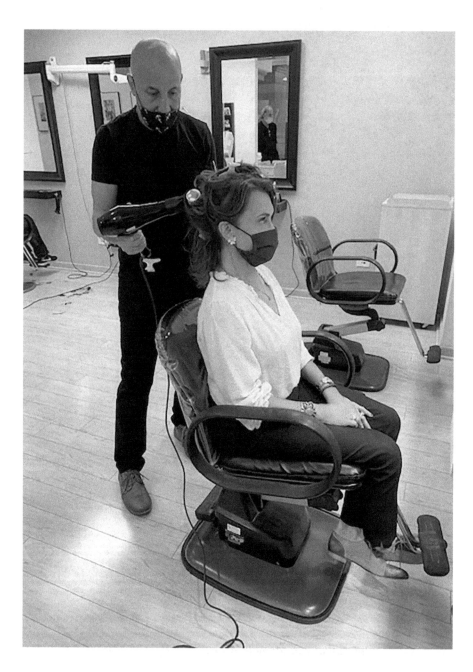

Personal care during a COVID-19 Life while
supporting a local business.

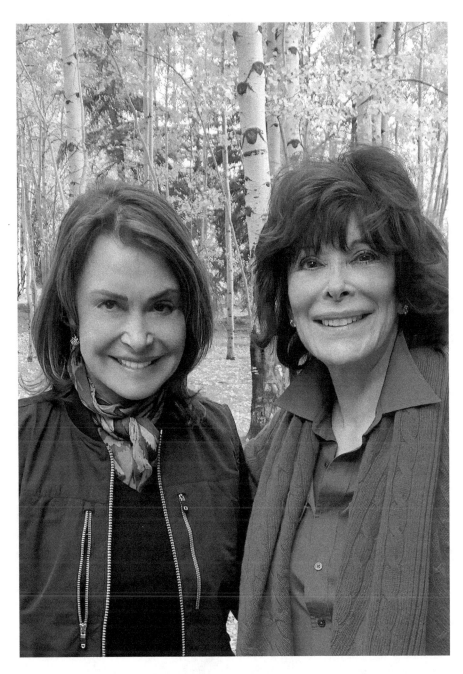

Pictured with Jill St. John who is the epitome of everlasting beauty taken in Aspen, which was my first post-COVID-lockdown travel destination.

CHAPTER 7

Vibrant Locks
(Best Practices, Diet,
and Going Gray)

Women do go bald, but they are better able to camouflage it than are men. Men are prone to bald patches, but women's hair thins. Thinning was starting to become a problem of mine. As I was looking into the matter, I came across that little bit of information.

There used to be an understanding that as a woman ages she should cut her hair and wear it short, because you just don't wear long hair as an older woman. Now that is untrue. There are older women who wear their hair long and look beautiful—Christie Brinkley and Cindy Crawford come to mind. They are in the entertainment world, but there are a lot of older women who wear their hair long and look wonderful.

Now there is a big "but" involved in deciding to wear your hair long. If you happen to have thin, straggly hair, then you should cut it fairly short. Holding onto your youthful looks by having long hair because it is appealing, sexy, and glamorous does not work if your hair is just not that thick and healthy looking.

Sustainable Tresses: Preventing and Recovering Hair Loss

Although it's common to lose anywhere from 50 to 100 strands of hair per day, for people with longer hair strands, losing them may be more noticeable. Hair loss also occurs because of stress, after giving birth, due to some diseases or medical treatments, for hereditary reasons, and most commonly, due to the aging process. According to the American Academy of Dermatology, "About 80 million men and women in the United States have this type of hair loss. . . . Luckily, most causes of hair loss can be stopped or treated."

With that in mind, and knowing that at some point, we will all go through this, I've put together a list of ways to prevent hair loss with some tips on what to do if you are already dealing with hair loss:

Visit your doctor, dermatologist, or hairdresser: At the first sign of hair loss, especially if it's sudden rather than gradual, you should consult with your doctor, dermatologist, and certainly your hairdresser, to determine any underlying factors. These professionals will be able to determine the cause and provide necessary treatment accordingly.

Topical treatments: In addition to following any advice provided by your healthcare or haircare professional, you can also try topical treatments that can be made at home. Here are some examples of homemade treatments:

- Boiling potatoes with rosemary and using the liquid as a rinse
- Mixing egg yolk and honey to use as a hair masque
- Brewing two bags of green tea in one cup of water and applying (once cool) to hair, leaving it in for one hour
- Adding aloe vera gel to your shampoo
- Mixing one tablespoon of lemon juice with two teaspoons of coconut or olive oil, and leaving mixture on scalp for one hour
- Rinsing hair with a combination of apple cider vinegar and warm water after washing

Massage: A daily hand massage on your scalp will help stimulate circulation while also stimulating hair follicles, keeping them active. Start near your forehead with your thumbs at your temples. Slowly begin to make firm pressure with your fingers as you move along the middle of your scalp. Extend outward with each pulse of your fingers, taking time to slowly massage every section. As a bonus, adding essential oils—like lavender, almond, rosemary or peppermint—provides an extra layer of aromatherapy, enhancing your overall well-being. Do this daily, for a few minutes, whenever possible.

Maintenance: Using a natural bristle brush will help stimulate hair follicles, increasing blood flow to the scalp. Make sure to brush your hair once it's dry or use a wide-tooth comb, gently, on wet hair. Letting your hair dry naturally instead of using a hot dryer also helps prevent hair loss and hair damage. The same applies for any heating tools you may use. Washing your hair in lukewarm—not hot—water prevents scalp and hair damage. And, try not to pull your hair into tight ponytails, buns, or braids, using soft methods instead.

Diet: In general, a well-balanced diet does your body good, so adding supplements like sources rich in protein and B vitamins, can help promote full and healthy hair. Try smoothies made with lettuce, capsicum, and carrots or spinach with berries and chia seeds. Vitamin C helps prevent breakage and brittle hair, so load up on oranges, guava, peppers, papaya, and dark leafy greens. And always make sure to drink plenty of liquids to keep your entire body, from head to toe, hydrated and replenished.

Foods for Healthy Hair

It's safe to say that everyone dreams of having long, thick, healthy hair. Our hair can be our proudest feature, and our pride shows with just how much maintenance we put into hair care. We wash, condition, and detangle it. We apply masques and treatments meant to moisturize, repair, strengthen, and define. We spend hours blow-drying, straightening, and styling it, and spend hundreds of dollars at salons every year to keep up with different services.

However, one thing is for sure—there's no amount of deep conditioners, masques, or trims that can make up for an unhealthy diet when it comes to hair growth. The things we put into our bodies is our first and most important method of nourishing our body, hair, and skin, because hair grows from within. Hair that is dry, brittle, frizzy, and weak, despite constant use of hair products, is usually a result of a bad diet.

It's important to remember that the macronutrients and micronutrients that our hair receives through our diet cannot always be supplied using topical products. A healthy diet that contains enough protein and healthy fats is the cornerstone of healthy hair. Here's what you should be eating often to ensure strong, healthy hair with remarkable growth.

Fatty Acids

Anyone who has ever told you that all forms of fat are bad is completely wrong. This isn't to say that the ten-piece bucket of fried chicken should be a staple in your diet, but good fats like omega-3s are major hair boosters, in terms of both growth and health. For shiny, lustrous hair that remains moisturized, try adding these foods that are high in good fats to your diet at least once a day:

- **Fatty fish:** Tuna, mackerel, salmon, and other types of fatty fish are great for you—and they taste great, too! Pan-sear a slice of fish as your main protein for dinner or lunch, and have it with vegetables as a filling meal. Tuna salad with a low-fat mayo can also be the perfect spread for a tasty sandwich, and you can even use the mix for a more low-carb vegetable dip.

- **Nuts:** Walnuts and almonds, for example, make for a healthy snack that can be eaten at any time to curb hunger and satiate your appetite.

Bananas, Spinach, and Potatoes

These foods are all high in vitamin B6. B-complex vitamins are all major components of healthy hair, as they strengthen hair to prevent splitting and breakage. For vitamin B12, meat and dairy products like cheese, milk, chicken, fish, and beef are all great sources.

Fruits and Veggies

Fruits and veggies are always welcome for a healthy body, and the same goes for hair. Citrus fruits, beans, and grains, as well as tomatoes, are high in folic acid, which helps to prevent thinning.

Protein

Protein is a no-brainer when it comes to healthy hair, as the hair is made of protein. More lean meats like chicken and fish are recommended, while eggs, beans, and soy products can make up a good part of your breakfast, lunch, and dinner options as well.

Having long healthy hair can be made so much simpler just by eating right. Add the right foods to your diet, eat them consistently, and don't overeat. Your body and hair will thank you.

Mayonnaise

Sometime in 1756, the French chef of Duke de Richelieu invented mayonnaise. Then the Romans made a fine mixture of eggs and olive oil, and this became known as the first real mayonnaise ever made.

We know mayo as that creamy lovely spread. It's tasty and is easily found in your kitchen. But have you ever wondered if mayo could do more than make a tasty snack? Some beauty experts would say that anything good enough to go down your tummy might just be good enough for the skin and hair—but be sure to do some research before trying to bathe in jam or all sorts of edible stuff.

Here are some benefits mayonnaise can offer in the beauty industry:

- **Hair conditioner:** By just thinking about it, you can see how your hair might benefit from a mayo conditioner, especially considering the main ingredients—egg and oil. To take advantage of this mayo benefit in skincare, massage a generous amount of mayo into your scalp and hair. Cover with a shower cap and leave it to sit for up to an hour. Wash off afterward for stronger, shinier, healthy hair.

- **Hydrated, soft skin:** Who would not want their skin to be baby soft? Simply lather on mayonnaise in a moderate amount and leave for about 10 minutes. Wash off and marvel at the soft, hydrated skin. The same method applies to a spa-worthy face masque.
- **Calms inflammation:** For inflammations like a sunburn situation, mayonnaise helps to calm things down and moisturize the skin. Apply mayonnaise liberally on the inflamed area and wash off later.

Rock Your Hair Color! (and Avoid the Pitfalls)

Hair coloring can be a tough process regardless of whether you do it at home or in the hair salon. From the time required to its cost, and products that don't turn out as promised, a lot of mistakes can be made. This can affect not only the results you get from the hair coloring process, but your overall hair health as well.

The secret to the successful coloring of hair lies in the little things only experts know. So, to help you rock your colored hair in style and avoid all the pitfalls, here are top tips for hair coloring from the experts:

Forget the lady on the box. It's amazing how we all make this mistake. The model on the box is there to get you to buy the product, and that beautiful shade she has on might not be the shade you get after using that dye. In fact, hair colorists say that the colors are always lighter than what you see on the package.

Don't dye all the way to the ends. Protect your ends and do not put the dye on them. Applying the hair color all the way to your ends can make them look heavy and inky.

Permanent or semi-permanent? Make a choice but choose wisely. If you opt for permanent hair color, pick a shade darker than what you want. The reason is, the developer in permanent dyes will lighten your hair. If you opt for semi-permanent dyes, pick a lighter shade than what you want. This is equally important because the longer it stays on, the darker the hair color becomes. These small adjustments help you get exactly what you are aiming for.

The way you do it matters. You might think all it takes to dye your hair is to slather on the color however you like, but that is a recipe for disaster. Hair color must be done in sections to avoid patchiness. First, section your hair vertically through the center of your forehead to the nape of your neck. Then do the same horizontally from one ear to the other. Tie up each section. Work from the back to the front to give the dye at the back of your hair enough time to set in. This makes the back darker just like your natural hair and gives you a natural look.

Use conditioner. When you have colored hair, a conditioner becomes an important beauty tool. First, during your root touch-ups, you can prevent your ends from getting stained by applying conditioner on them before washing. Also, conditioning your hair after coloring helps to keep it moisturized and closes the hair cuticles opened up by the dye. Hence, your shade won't go darker, and you can enjoy your colored hair as much as you like.

Tool up. Don't minimize the proper tools needed to dye your hair. Use a toothbrush for highlights, two mirrors, and quality dye. If you are going to the hair salon to get this done by a stylist, ensure they are expert colorists.

The Generous Guide to Going Gray

If you're thinking about going gray and finally allowing your salt-and-pepper strands to grow freely, the chances are that you're pretty nervous. However, there's good news! Letting your mane go gray doesn't have to be scary. With this simple guide on steps to make the process easier, you'll find that achieving glorious gray tresses isn't half as difficult as you imagined.

Fight the Stigma

You've surely seen it before – a woman panicking at the sight of her first gray hair. Gray hair is associated with getting older, and because getting older has been considered a negative change for the longest time, gray strands are targeted on sight.

Men and women both experience the fear of graying hair, but it's time to do away with the cover-ups, dyes, and plucking that often follows. By embracing the natural process of aging, you allow yourself to let go of society's beauty standards. Natural beauty is just as worthy as cosmetically-enhanced beauty, and it's time that the world knew it.

Make Salon Plans

Finding a competent hairdresser who knows what they're doing makes the journey to gray much easier. Will you choose to keep your natural gray color or blend it with natural-looking lowlights and highlights to enhance your hair's look? The final product lies in the hands of the hairstylist you choose to trust with your hair. Ensure that they are educated and experienced about the graying process and that they know exactly how to bring out the best in your locks.

Gradual Chops Can Save Your Life

If you've been leaving your roots to grow freely in preparation for an all-out gray mane, then there's great news! You won't have to wait for your roots to grow out. As your gray roots continue to grow, small chops every few months or twice a year can be the perfect way to get closer to a full head of gray without having to compromise much of your length.

If you don't mind rocking short hair and prefer a big chop to get directly to gray hair, you can opt for that route, too. The option you feel most comfortable with is the one you'll feel most confident with.

A Cut That Suits Your Face, Style, and Lifestyle Is Key

Gray hair can look bland without some sort of shape or cut to spice it up a bit. A cut that makes your gray hair pop is great to keep things interesting. It's up to you whether a short, medium-length, or long cut is best, of course!

There are no one-size-fits-all when it comes to the best cut for gray hair. You might love how a style looks quite different, but you may find that it looks very different on you. To avoid a cut that you can't undo, ensure that your hairstylist assesses your face shape, personal preferences, and lifestyle to help you make the best possible choice.

Color Crazy? Leave It to the Pros

If you decide to go the color route, there's one thing that you absolutely must avoid: trying to recreate the perfect silver tones yourself. Stylists do more than just apply a block of pigment to your hair. They're trained in where and how to apply the right lowlights and highlights to fit the shade of your hair.

Attempting to do the job yourself could mean a messy tragedy for the health and appearance of your hair. It's just not worth it to risk damaging your precious mane! Though a professional salon color job can be quite expensive, it's an investment in your looks that is sure to pay off.

The Right Hair Products Can Make or Break Your Hair!

Choosing to go gray comes with the need for more attention placed on the products that you'll be using. Gray and silver hair can tend to turn yellow or brassy-looking over time, especially if you've had it colored professionally. To avoid that old-newspaper look, you'll need to get your hands on the right products for your hair and ensure that you use them as consistently as they're required to be used.

Purple shampoo and conditioners and even purple rinses can help to keep that perfect silver hue for as long as possible. Whether your hair has been colored or is a natural silver/gray color, specially formulated products like these can make the biggest difference in maintaining your silver locks.

Own Your Look

Transitioning from your usual hair color to gray hair can be quite a shocker. You might feel uncomfortable at first— you might even feel like everyone's watching you or judging you! But the truth is this: There's nothing more beautiful and fulfilling than learning to accept your body for what it naturally does, grays and all.

Your graying hair is just as acceptable as any other hue. Finding ways to complement it can make you feel much more at ease. Gray hair has no color, so colorful clothes, makeup, or jewelry can be the perfect way to add some life into your look.

The journey to going fully gray is quite an experience. Sure, you'll learn a lot about your hair, but you'll learn a lot about yourself, too. You'll see your gray hair as a crown, as a gentle reminder of the years that you've lived through and made the most of. Getting older isn't a punishment, it's a blessing. Letting your gray strands take over with this handy guide will surely be a breeze.

Hair Today, Gone Tomorrow

One of the reasons why women do lose their hair is because of the impact of shampooing on the oils and cuticle in the scalp. It is not a good idea to shampoo your hair every day, and some women do. Some shampoo every other day, and some once a week. Regardless, for a more mature woman, I would suggest using a shampoo that is actually not a shampoo, but a co-wash or a cleansing conditioner, which is sulfate-free. "Co-wash" means conditioning washing, and it is a product designed to be milder than shampoo, not stripping away the natural oils as the surfactants in shampoo would do. As I mentioned earlier, I did try this even though I was reluctant because it was hard to imagine how it would get my hair clean. And then, I realized how much nicer using a co-wash product makes my hair look, much thicker.

The reason long hair looks good on a younger person is generally because it is thicker. The volumizing shampoos are quite bad and drying on the hair, so I strongly suggest staying away from those. Of course, hair dye and a lot of other things you may do to your hair to make yourself look better is going to be a detriment for your hair as well.

One thing I had been trying to work on with my hair stylist is that I like my hair being streaked, as do many women. Especially for older women, a little light around the face makes you look better. She said, "Hey, instead of lightening your hair around the temples, why don't we start lower and then put the base of your color a little lighter each time? So it's a gradual transition. You won't see the gray, and you won't have to do it as often."

That was a good tip. And it is a style that has a name—*balayage*. That is where you start streaking your hair much lower than they used to do for normal highlighting up at the root area. The color is hand-painted on and results in natural looking highlights. It requires less maintenance partly because it is designed to look as if the roots had grown out. So I started doing this, and it has been very helpful. For me, trying something like this comes down to the caliber of my stylist, whom I fully trust.

CHAPTER 8

Style after 60

Eyebrows play such a big part in the appearance of a woman's face. As I mentioned, my mother didn't have eyebrows, and for her entire life, she had to pencil them in. She always reminded me, "You're so lucky to have eyebrows." As I got older, I started going balder on my eyebrows, and I would wonder, *Do I tattoo my eyebrows?* Because that was a big thing. Yet, I was frightened to death to do that because I have a major scar in my eyebrow from my car accident. I thought, *If I tattoo and my skin drops down a little bit, with the tattoo staying high, what the hell would that look like?*

So I did a little further research, and of course, microblading was becoming a big thing. But I was pretty hesitant as the method used didn't sound all that appealing. That technique is where they scrape your eyebrow and deposit a little color. It is done by a highly trained hand, and in a fashion where you can hardly tell it's been done.

I gave it more thought and looked into it further. I found someone who came highly recommended. The gal I found began talking to me about it and said, "Just come in and I'll explain it to you." So I did. I explained to her my concerns and how it would be her challenge to try and color the part of my eyebrow that was scarred. To women out there who have had similar problems, this is absolutely for them. But only with the right stylist because the color does not react on scar tissue the same as it would on regular tissue. I had many questions, which she answered, and so I chose to try it.

Simple Routines for Staying Stylish

I am often asked how I stay stylish after 60. The truth is . . . I am over 70. As women grow older, they become particularly skittish about expressing themselves with style. Sometimes it's because they are self-conscious, while other times it's simply because they just don't know how to go about styling themselves to look good.

In my opinion, staying stylish is as easy as it gets! With a few simple and routine steps, any female over 60 can look as stylish as she wants. In fact, several designers have stylish fashion trends suitable for both young and older women so there's no reason for any woman to not look beautiful, regardless of her age.

Here are five winning tips you shouldn't ignore, and I hope they help you take that next step in feeling and looking stylish:

1. **YOUR SMILE**

   A beautiful smile is timeless and works wonders in more ways than can be imagined. This is why it's critical that every woman pay attention to her dental health. In addition to regularly brushing and flossing, a visit to a cosmetic dentist can also help brighten a smile with moderate whitening, as well as fixing any tooth irregularities.

2. **GREAT FOOTWEAR**

   For most women, footwear may seem like nothing but donning the right shoe, but it can go a long way in improving your appearance. There are now comfortable shoes in every style—from kitten heels and flats and even flip-flops to sling-back heels. And remember, these fashionable shoes will look great on well-groomed legs and stylishly manicured feet.

3. **FITNESS**

   Although working out is great, one must be careful to not overdo it so you don't end up appearing overly taut, toned, or even haggard looking. Staying fit is a must but don't push things to the extreme. Keep active every day with simple things like a morning walk, light cycling, stretching, and even yoga. And rest! Make sure there's enough rest at the end of your day to replenish your energy for the next day.

4. STRAY GRAYS

For some over 60, looking stylish means keeping the gray far and away. Talk to your beautician or stylist and ask to go through different hues and textures to see which hairstyle suits you best. It's great to experiment with color if it makes you feel beautiful.

5. GREAT LIPS

We tend to forget about our lips and how to keep them youthful, plump, and rejuvenated, especially when it comes to color. Aside from using a hydrating moisturizer or balm, it's important to pay attention to color.

Best Lipstick Colors for Women over 50

Society has made people believe that women start to lose their beauty as they grow older. However, this couldn't be any further from the truth. We believe that a beautiful woman never loses track of her charm even when she hits her fifties, especially if she grooms herself and accessorizes her looks with the right kind of makeup, jewelry, and clothes.

When it comes to fashion, lipstick is one of the main things that showcase your nature. As time goes by, you have to change your range of lip colors to suit your age group and status. For the ladies who have hit their fifties, we have compiled a list of lip colors that would best suit women over 50.

Maroon: Never let anyone tell you to step away from bold colors just because you're growing older. With strong shades like maroon, burgundy, and wine, you can never go wrong in showcasing your evergreen and bold charm.

Peach: There's nothing like a soft, peachy pink shade to decorate your look when you're feeling especially girly and carefree, since this lip color will make you look just as young as you feel.

Mauve: When you think of the color mauve, what comes to your mind is sophistication and professionalism, both of which are traits all ladies over 50 want to portray while stepping in to work or even just dinner with some colleagues.

Perfect Makeup Right Out of Bed!

Don't let anyone tell you that being 50 means you should put a lid on your love for makeup. No matter what age you are, you should never stop experimenting with colors. You just have to find the right shades for yourself, and now that you have our list of best lipsticks for women over 50, you can easily choose the right color to showcase your personality.

Have you ever wished you could get out of bed, primed and ready to go? Of course, we have all wished for that. Waking up to perfectly set eyebrows, full juicy lips, blackened shiny lashes, and a bright complexion doesn't seem like too much to ask for. Yet in the past, ladies have had to settle for hours at the dressing table achieving each of these and more.

Yes, such time-consuming and unnerving days can quickly get buried in the past with an emerging trend called semi-permanent makeup.

One good thing about advancement in technology and product manufacturing is how they strive to meet your unique needs. The continued desire for effortlessly good-looking skin and a ready-to-go appearance has gotten gears shifting and labs churning to provide solutions. Hence, semi-permanent makeup has become a thing and as far as a description goes, it is exactly what it sounds like. It is a collection of advanced technologies that apply natural-looking makeup just so you can wake up the way you have always dreamed.

How it works, depends on what you want or need. Here are some brands offering these new developments.

For filtered skin, check out the new procedure from Korea known as BB Glow. BB Glow involves a treatment with lots of tiny needles, serums, and pigments to give you a natural-looking filtered skin. It is a one-off procedure of nano-needling, giving you the results you want. They last for a few weeks before fading away. The treatments cost $550 each.

There are benefits to semi-permanent makeup such as a time- and money-saving, youthful appearance, as well as an end to the struggle for perfectly applied makeup. For some, that last benefit trumps everything and is worth trying all these procedures and the latest innovations. Oh, the struggle of waking up each morning to stubborn eyebrows, and then spending hours trying to get them in perfect shape. Sometimes after all your hard work, you stand back and look in the mirror only to find that you did not ace the shape at all. Urgh!

If it's any comfort, this is the daily routine for most ladies, except if you are a celebrity who has long invested in getting the perfect eyebrows tattooed on her skin. Yet, the fact is, the trend is growing. Perhaps soon, it won't be so strange to always look like you have perfect makeup on, and when your friends ask, you can just go, "Yes, it's semi-permanent makeup. I got everything last week."

Microblading—Eyebrows Perfected

Microblading is a procedure that has the entire beauty industry buzzing. On one hand, it seems like a dream come true for every female because, after all, who wouldn't want to wake up to perfect eyebrows. But on the other hand, it seems sketchy too. The words tattoo, ink, and needles may have you thinking twice. So what is microblading, and is it worth it? Well, you can answer those questions after getting fully informed.

What is microblading?

Microblading is a beauty technique that involves the use of a precise tool to deposit pigment into the skin. Some refer to this tool as a super-fine pen containing up to fifteen needles. The tips are so fine that they create accurate hair strokes to blend with your eyebrow hairs. Unlike other techniques, microblading can simulate hair and has the most natural look.

Does it hurt?

A little, yes.

What is the procedure?

The entire procedure usually takes about 30 to 40 minutes, sometimes an hour. You should arrive at an appointment on time. The eyebrow specialist will consult with you about the best shape for your eyebrow. When that's settled, the specialist will proceed to outline the shape. A numbing agent will be used to numb the area and reduce any pain. Then, your eyebrow specialist will get to work implanting featherweight strokes. If you start to feel discomfort, more numbing ointment will be applied. Most times, you can keep checking your eyebrows until you love what you see. The entire process is careful and sterile.

Is it pricey?

Sure it is. Microblading takes its worth in money by being quite pricey. Prices can range from $400 to $800, with the average procedure costing around $600.

What happens next?

There is a follow-up session after six to eight weeks to be sure you love your brows and there are no problems. There are a few rules to follow after microblading:

- No makeup for at least a week
- Use sunscreen to increase the longevity of the brows and protect from the sun
- Do not get the brows wet for a week

Following these rules helps the brows to heal faster and get settled for you to enjoy your splurge.

How long does it last?

Depending on your skin type, the microblading technique gives you eyebrows that last from one to three years. You can touch up after twelve months so they don't fade away.

What do I think?

Well, who would pass up the opportunity to wake up looking like a lady indeed? Microblading equals stress-free eyebrows, and if you are scared of needles, remember the numbing agent is there for you.

Microblading for Men

Like brow microblading, scalp microblading is a temporary tattooing procedure that embeds cosmetic pigments into the dermis (unlike a permanent tattoo where ink is deposited below the dermis). The idea is to recreate natural-looking strokes that replicate the appearance of real hair and conceal any thinning areas on the scalp.

This particular microblading process involves artfully blending tattooed strokes with your natural hair, so you're more likely to recreate the realistic effect of a lush, healthy mane in areas where you still have hair growth. If your hair loss is more severe with larger bald patches, scalp microblading may not be your best bet.

Your Evolving Beauty Regimen

Beauty tips change along with your age; therefore, it's hard to keep up with the ever-changing dos and don'ts of makeup when it comes to retaining your youth. As soon as you've passed your 50s, it's necessary to change up your skincare and makeup routine that you had at a time when you didn't have to worry about wrinkles, fine lines, and age spots. This is why I compiled a brand new beauty routine that will become your partner in helping you look youthful and full of life.

Makeup and Beauty Tips

#1 A Moisturizing Primer Is Your Best Friend

I cannot stress enough the importance of moisturizing your skin before applying makeup as it reduces the appearance of fine lines and immediately makes your skin look fresher. For that, I recommend using a moisturizing primer.

#2 Avoid Piling up on Powder

Due to the fact that wrinkles and fine lines often appear as you grow older, applying powder ends up making your face look cakey and overdone. I recommend using a thin and subtle concealer and foundation, and then finishing your look off with a setting spray that instead will make your skin glow, which is a big requirement for a younger appearance.

#3 Use a Volumizing Mascara

A volumizing mascara will make your eyes appear fuller and childlike, instantly giving you a young, fresh, and active look.

Once you have this flawless base with the help of these tips and tricks, your skin will look youthful and vibrant in no time because a healthy skincare routine is the first step in the process of anti-aging. Remember ladies, your skin always comes first!

As you grow older, your skin requires different products than we used in our teens, 20s or 30s. With time your skin decreases the production of collagen which makes the skin sag faster and look wrinkled. However, all these aging symptoms can be hidden with the use of proper makeup products that are made specifically for mature skin. If you want to take a few years off your face with the help of makeup and beauty tricks, you have come to the right place. Here are a few tips and tricks that you can use every day for flawless and youthful-looking skin.

#1 Use Lip and Cheek Tint

100-Percent Pure Fruit Pigmented Lip and Cheek Tint
Instead of using a powder blush that can accentuate
the fine lines on your skin, go for a gentle lip and
cheek tint that is in a liquid form. It gives a natural,
rosy color to your complexion and makes your skin
look youthful.

#2 Go for a Liquid Highlighter

Drugstore Liquid Highlighter
You can totally skip highlighter for everyday makeup.
A liquid highlighter gives you a dewy and natural
glow that makes your skin look young and healthy.

#3 Avoid Harsh Colors

Sharply contoured red lips and stark-black eyeliner
sound appealing, but all this can add years to your face.
Stick to a brown eyeliner to look naturally beautiful.

With these makeup and beauty tips up your sleeve, you
will be able to look young and beautiful effortlessly. Adopt
these expert tips and make all the heads turn with your
timeless beauty.

Eyebrows Perfected? The Verdict Is In

Finally the day came to have my microblading done. I went
and I was just terrified sitting in the seat waiting to have
this done. It reminded me of when I was considering some
sort of surgery to my eyes, many moons ago, because they

are a little unbalanced. A couple of surgeons with whom I'd consulted told me, "This is what we do. We take your face and divide it into four sections: top left and right, bottom left and right. Your eyebrows are the center point most people see first. If they are unbalanced in any way, your face seems a little distorted." Now that being said, this is a good test: take a picture of your left side profile and your right side profile. When you try to put them together, it can appear to be two different faces.

So there I was. First, they numb your eyebrows, and then, they use these little blades and cut tiny scrapes, where they deposit color. That is definitely not a tattoo because it is not permanent, only semi-permanent. I looked in the mirror and absolutely freaked out. I looked like Groucho Marx. "What is this?!" I said. She replied, "Don't worry, that's what it looks like now. It is just a bit of color deposited. In a few hours, I will wipe away most of it." I had no choice, so I took her word for it.

Well, in any event, when she did wipe them down, I said, "Oh, they're okay. But still a little thick." She told me, "Just don't touch anything. Wait a couple of days and it will be exactly what you want." Lo and behold, she was right. They turned out perfect. I was so happy. This might be one of the best procedures I've had done, the most successful. You get these teeny scabs, but when you put a little vitamin E on it, they quickly disappear. I have been back for touch ups, and plan to continue doing so. So I say this to women who are thinking of getting this procedure and are frightened of it:

Go ahead and do it if it is something you want to do. Having been through it, I do advocate it.

So other than the hair on my head disappearing and my eyebrows as well, there is the matter of pubic hair. These are all part of the natural aging process, but it doesn't go well for some women. Women are always concerned about how they look, and the hair under the arms, on the legs, the pubic hair are all signs of sexuality. When these things disappear, even though women may not speak about it, they do think about it. So you do what you can to address these changes, and I do fully recommend this procedure.

CHAPTER 9

Makeup
(Skin, Eyes, and
Maintaining Your Kit)

For a long time following my auto accident, I didn't think about makeup. Matter of fact, the last thing on my mind was makeup. But as my healing progressed, I began exploring how I was going to cover these scars on my face. I did endless research and what I found out is that there was a lot of bad makeup out there.

I went on a quest to find a truly good makeup, one that would actually cover the scars. In my search, I met a makeup artist by the name of Art Anthony, who made prostheses for different actors—extra noses or different kinds of ears, flawless skin to cover bad acne, and things of that nature. So I asked him to help me find a makeup to cover my scars, and he did. He tried very hard to help me, but it was all too thick and gooey to do the job. So I did some reconnaissance on how to get them covered up.

One lucky thing for me was that all my scars were on one side of my face. So I was able to train my hair to fall on one side, using a side part. It took me a good year to get it trained, as I had parted it before either in the middle or the opposite side. Finally, it came to fall correctly, lying down in a way where it did cover the scars. So that was one of my methods for concealing them.

At the time, I was still modeling, but of course, it was pretty limited. I had to totally stay away from certain angles on the camera because my face just looked weird. And even though I was able to shield that area and take certain angles looking up or down, keeping it going for me, I needed to go back to the chalkboard and find a good foundation. I needed just the right color in just the right shade, and to learn how to make it work on my face. As time passed, I worked with the very best makeup artists. They all taught me a bunch of tricks, and eventually, I was able to find a decent makeup.

The most essential trick I learned is that *less is more.* The trick came down to finding a balance in having the right amount of makeup on to cover the scars, without looking pasty or sick. Sometimes, people even said, "Wow, you look great, and without makeup." In fact, I was wearing tons of makeup. So it is a skill to be able to put on a lot of makeup and have it look as if you are wearing next to none. I learned to do that and it paid off for me. I became so happy about that and my choices. I always tried to look vibrant, and for the most part, I think I accomplished that.

Beauty and Makeup Tips for Flawless-Looking Skin

Everyone wants to achieve flawless skin. Some improve their skincare game, and some master the skills of makeup to have that flawless-looking skin. But in this era, it is a must to balance both skincare and makeup to show off your perfect skin.

Here are a few tips on how to achieve flawless looking skin with the help of proper skincare and makeup techniques:

- **Exfoliating Your Skin Is A Must:** Our skin sheds itself on a daily basis. However, in that process, some parts of our dry and dead skin fail to shed and clog our pores. To make sure no dead skin is left, exfoliate your skin thrice a week. This step will help you get a smooth canvas for your makeup application.
- **Primer Is Your Best Friend:** Always prime your skin to create a barrier between your skin and the makeup. Not all ingredients used in the makeup products are perfect for your skin. The primer also helps in applying the makeup smoother than ever.
- **Never Skip Sunscreen:** It is a major misconception that sunscreen is for summers only. No matter what the weather, it is necessary to put on some sunscreen to help your skin stay protected from the harmful UVA and UVB rays.
- **Less Is Always More:** When applying makeup, always keep in mind that less product is always more.

Generously applying makeup can make your skin look cakey and unnatural instantly.

- **Double Cleanse Your Skin:** After a whole day of wearing makeup and exposing your skin to all the pollutants in our environment, your skin needs to be deeply cleansed. Use an oil-based cleanser to take off all your makeup, followed by a foaming cleanser to make your skin squeaky clean.

With these quick and easy tips, you will be able to achieve the skin that you have always wanted without compromising on makeup.

Best Eyeshadow Colors for Women over 50

A lot of mature women avoid eyeshadow and sometimes any makeup at all. It's not that they don't want to add color and enhance their best features with a good ole makeup session. The problem is that the makeup industry is rather ageist.

Well, a revolution in this area seems quite far away, but thankfully, you can make do with the right tips and an upgrade to your beauty routine.

Now, the toughest part about finding the best makeup for older women is that we need products that don't smudge, smear, and flake, or worse, move into the fine lines. We need makeup that helps to bring out the best versions of our older selves, not making us appear like an old dame desperately clinging to her youth.

There are several factors that come into play to give you the best makeup for mature skin. Read on to learn them all:

Eyeshadow Colors

Colors play a vital role in makeup. They determine how everything sits on your skin, giving you the look you desire. First, you need a product that doesn't flake or smear; matte palettes are a great option.

Soft and neutral colors favor mature women more than anything. Try to forget about how you rocked that black stuff around the eyes, and think only of colors that match your skin tone. Colors like gray, taupe, cream, are suitable for anyone.

Bright eyeshadows make your eyes look dramatic. Especially with hooded eyes. Dark eyeshadows make your eyes seem smaller. So you want to avoid both bright and dark eyeshadows. Natural and light-colored shadows make your eyes pop, looking vibrant, and youthful. It makes your eyes the focus of your face and outshines those wrinkles and fine lines.

The way to do this is to apply any pale eyeshadow, and then use a complementary darker shade to form a fine line along the lash line. Don't panic if your application isn't perfect. Focus on pushing the dark color to the base of the lashes, and then use a brush to sweep it up at the outer edge.

This can easily become a dependable routine to make the right colors work for you. Here is a way to match colors:

- Cream and cocoa brown
- Pale gray and charcoal gray
- Taupe and dark green or a dark purple

Always Apply a Primer

A primer can serve as the best foundation for mature skin. Prime your face, but most importantly, your eyelids before makeup. It helps to reduce the visible signs of aging and keep the makeup put on the eyes all day.

Curl Your Lashes

After all your hard work on getting the right colors for mature skin to pop, you must curl your lashes. This is like the icing on the cake. It wraps up your eye makeup by adding volume, length, and shape to your lashes.

Brows

When you are in your 50s or higher, brows can thin out, making it hard to achieve a complete look. Feel confident to fill out your thin brows. Do this artfully and lightly. They can be thin, but make them seen.

How to Clean Your Makeup Brushes

You should be shocked to learn that most women hardly clean their makeup brushes as they should. But you are not because, at some point, we are all guilty!

Makeup brushes are just about the most essential of makeup tools because, without them, your routine would be a sloppy mess. So, we dab and apply with these brushes every day, without ever thinking of getting them cleaned. Or we think about it, but just decide we don't have the time. The thing is, this is bad news for your skin because of the buildup of product and bacteria on those brushes.

The consequences of daily grime include skin irritation, breakouts, and congestion. Let's not forget that clogged bristles won't work as well either, and that can be frustrating.

Read on as we discuss how to clean makeup brushes:

Cleaning Makeup Brushes

STEPS

1. Set all your brushes aside from the rest of your makeup
2. Get a glass or mug (deep enough for you to work with) and fill with warm water
3. Add a dollop of shampoo to the water
4. Place the brushes in and swirl them in the water
5. Bring them out one at a time to massage the bristles and slough off deep-seated gunk
6. Your brushes should turn the color they were before getting covered in product
7. Rinse with clean water and lay them out to dry, without clumping together

How often should you clean your brushes? Every week! Yes, once a week is the minimum number of times to wash your brushes.

Best Brush Hygiene Tips

- For brushes or blenders used to apply liquid products, clean more often. At least three to four times per week will do to prevent the buildup of organisms like fungi and bacteria that thrive in moist environments.
- Opt for synthetic brushes. Synthetic brushes last longer and are easy to clean. Natural brushes tend to get worn out easily especially if you do not clean them. Natural bristles are also porous, which makes these brushes high maintenance and expensive in the long run.
- Always store your makeup brushes in cool and dry places. Store them separately from other tools.
- Avoid leaving brushes in damp areas that could attract bacteria.
- Air dry your makeup brushes and blenders often.
- Synthetic brushes usually clump together when there is too much gunk from product buildup. Fluffy or natural brushes pile up products at their base, indicating it's time for a clean.

How do you know when it's time to replace?

Some ladies wait until the brushes simply won't cooperate anymore. This is unhealthy for your skin, frustrating, and most times, unexpected. If your makeup brushes start to shed or no longer work for you, then it is a sure sign replacement is needed. Other signs include holding on to stains after cleaning. Makeup experts advise that you buy a few new brushes periodically. This is a healthy and cost-effective way to replace makeup brushes.

Makeup Storage Tips

I don't know about you, but to me, nothing feels more satisfying than having an organized makeup closet. I have learned it makes it easier to perform your beauty routine on time and keep everything clean and fresh.

If you can't seem to keep your makeup organized for more than a day, then you are in luck. Read on as I dish out practical makeup storage tips to help you stay at the top of your game.

PS: If you are a makeup minimalist, you probably have few makeup products, all of which would fit in one box. As long as you maintain them properly, you will be fine. These tips below are for makeup junkies—ladies with more products than they even use.

- **Separate Your Makeup Brushes:** Makeup brushes are a vital part of everyday makeup. The best way to store them neatly and properly is to separate them from other makeup items. Place all your brushes in a cup or glass jar. Place the jar on the countertop or a clean and dust-free area.

- **Clear Plastic:** Trust me, I am just like you; I usually throw out any plastic wrapping that comes with my makeup. But when it came down to keeping things organized, I realized those plastic wraps can do much more. Store your eyeshadow quads in a clear plastic pouch. If you can't get these wraps, then purchase plastic containers just like them. Use them to keep your loose makeup items together so they stay organized.

- **Favorites:** Which products do you use more often? Separate these daily favorites from the rest and store them in a makeup bag or box in a super accessible location. When you think about it, you realize that searching for the products you use frequently usually leads to messing up your makeup closet.

- **Jewelry Box for Lipsticks:** Get an old jewelry box and set all your lipsticks in it with the color sides facing up. This makes it easier to identify the color you want, pull it out, use it, and push it back in. Fix the problem of littering lipsticks across your bathroom counter with this tip.

- **Put Vintage Plates to Work:** Old dinnerware can do more than sit abandoned in the kitchen cupboard. Show off these pieces by using them to hold your makeup items. Choose suitable sizes that can store your products while keeping them dust-free.

- **Makeup drawers:** Makeup drawers are a great storage option. You can purchase different designs and sizes from most makeup stores. Keep the items you need or use often in the drawer closest to you and organize others accordingly.

Remember the key is to make all your items accessible but in a dust- and dirt-free environment. Pull this off for longer than 24 hours and it should stick as a habit.

A Wedding Day Dream Come True

On the day of your wedding, you want your makeup, your look, and just everything about you to be perfect. I was not a young bride. I got married after turning 70. Pretty amazing in itself! But it took all the tricks of the trade in the things that I consistently did to make that day a success. So here is something that turned out to be surprising about this for me: I had two weddings! My first wedding was in July, and totally by surprise. You could say I was shocked.

My husband-to-be, Arny, and I were visiting Venice, Italy, which long has been one of his favorite places. He had wanted to take me there for some time. So finally, we arrived, and it was a rather casual place. Knowing that, I hadn't brought any fancy clothes with me. But that night, he said to me, "Why don't you get a little dressed up tonight, and maybe we'll have an extra special celebration of life."

So that sounded fine. I took a look through my wardrobe, where I found a pretty short mini-dress with fringe hanging down. A real sixties look. My hair wasn't particularly done, so I put it in a ponytail. I scurried around for some makeup that I'd tossed in my purse, which worked out well. Then, I headed downstairs to meet him in the lobby.

Well, waiting for me in the lobby with Arny was a gondolier, who told me, "Your gondola awaits you."

When we got to the gondola, there was a big bouquet of flowers, which he handed me. I still wasn't sure what was going on, but we started traveling down the canal. And we came across this beautiful building from another century, just gorgeous. Standing at the bottom of the stairs was a man, someone like a justice of the peace, and he said, "Are you ready to get married?" I looked at Arny, and said, "Are you kidding me?" He answered, "Yes, we're getting married tonight."

Of course, someone had to just about pick me up from the floor. But we walked up the stairs of this beautiful castle—yes, it really was a castle. And there were all these violinists from the Venetian Orchestra playing violins. We walked through this marble entrance to a big desk, where there were two large seats as if for a king and queen. And he married us. We handed the girl who was there our iPhone, and she took a little video of the wedding.

Now mind you, this would be the most important day in most women's lives. I was there wearing my mini-dress with my hair in a ponytail. I was thinking a little of how I was going to look back for years at my wedding day. Well it all worked out fine. We got back in the gondola, and as we were streaming down the canals, people were throwing rose petals over the bridges. It looked like a scene out of George Clooney's wedding. Just like that. And there was the man standing at the back of the gondola swishing that big oar back and forth, singing and whistling the wedding song. It was so different and so romantic.

We ended up at a place on the other side of the island called L'Alcova Restaurant, where we had our wedding dinner. There we were, he and I and a big bottle of champagne. And so, we proceeded to have a pretty good time. I was still in shock, and just couldn't believe it. Arny had arranged for a photographer, who would bounce around from one bridge to another. Every time we passed under a bridge, there was the photographer. He was like Peter Pan. He was just shooting pictures like crazy.

So after all that wonderful preparation and everything being said, we learned upon getting back to the States that we were not actually married. All the paperwork had to be in 17 days before, and his was in 16 days. So Arny said, "Well, we either leave it like that, or we get married in Chicago." So we had another wedding, inviting 350 people. A big blast at Arny's country club, Oak Park Country Club. And on that day, I was totally prepared.

A bride's dress was a big thing in my mind. I wondered, at my age do I wear a long white dress with a veil? I was certainly not a virgin. In any event, I pulled it off. The dress was gorgeous, and I am so glad I did that. I was so excited. Arny picked out the music, "You Are So Beautiful" by Joe

Cocker. As I walked down the aisle, there wasn't a dry eye in the place because I am blessed by so many people in my life, good friends who love me. And so, the ceremony took place and it was magical.

I had my bridesmaids (some who had come in from Europe), and we all had photos taken. It was so very nice. I remember looking in the mirror and thinking, "Well, I guess my years of discipline and consistency in my regimen paid off." I had a big smile on my face, and I thought that I did look beautiful, if I must say. Everything was about a bride and groom having a day that was so beautiful in their lives. I was so very happy that day.

My husband is also a magician, not by trade, more of a hobby. With this in mind . . . Instead of having your traditional wedding, he and I popped out of a box, a wedding box called *the book of love*, and then he made me disappear. And all of a sudden, I reappeared to the audience. The same thing with the justice of the peace. He disappeared and appeared, and I didn't quite know how he did this. Everybody was like, *Oh, my God!*

At the end, instead of having a big wedding cake, everybody had a cupcake with their name on it. It was pretty cool. I loved sharing this day with my family and friends. Though, there was one very special friend missing that day. That was Suzanne, who was not able to make it.

And now, I am trying to get through life with all of the craziness going on in the world, grateful for my good friends and for Arny, as we go on celebrating our union.

CHAPTER 10

A Joyful Life
with Animals

Tranquility, peace, and a grand sense of well-being are all the things I feel when I ride my horse. I grew up in the city and have lived there my entire life. Generally, when you live in the city, it's unlikely you would own a horse. When I was eleven years old, there was an amusement park that had horses, both the merry-go-round horses and the real ones. I went to the park to ride on the rides, but when I saw the horses, I decided to give riding them a try. It was love at first ride!

I felt so happy on that horse that I went back twice a week for years. I was very young at the time. I would take a bus and ride at least an hour, and then walk a couple of miles to the amusement park where you could ride. This went on for quite some time. As a young adult, I started advancing into horse jumping and joining these small shows, as well as doing a little show jumping.

With horses, it is like anything else—you keep learning and graduating into bigger and better skills. You start with a walk, then go to a trot, a cantor, a gallop, and then you go on to a jump. It is a natural transition. But you do need to have each of those skills down before you move on to the next level. And when you become so efficient and are riding your horse so well, like anything else, you want more challenges. You buy a car you like, and eventually you find yourself buying an even nicer car. You finish reading a terrific book, which inspires you to educate yourself further so you get a more advanced book. Same thing with horses.

I wanted to own my own horse, so I went horse shopping and purchased my first horse when I was fifteen. Who would have thought I could own my own horse? My horse taught me so many things. As I was growing with my relationship to my horse during those years, it taught me discipline and responsibility. And today, my goal is to own my own horse farm.

One thing I love about riding horses is the way it is like skiing. While riding, it's just you and the animal. While skiing, it's just you and your mountain. When you play tennis, you have to have a partner. But with riding, you become one with your horse. And you learn pretty fast in the process that horses do indeed have a brain. Horses are disciplined. They can learn. But they are large creatures and they can cause pain as well. One must always stay alert when on the back of a horse. It is a great feeling, rather powerful in itself. Still, these are large animals, and they can be a bit unpredictable. So you don't want to be too relaxed on them.

I've watched many shows on TV about other riders and other related disciplines like dressage, show jumping, cross-country, and the rodeo. It's always fun to watch the barrel riders; they are pretty tough riders. For me, I'll stick to hunters & jumpers. While I was riding, I came across a sport that was truly fascinating to me—fox hunting.

The hunt tradition has gone on since the 1500s in Europe, England, Ireland, and Scotland. I have ridden horses and hunted on horses worldwide. The guidelines vary in each country and community. In my community, they do a replica tradition of the hunt, meaning there is no actual fox involved.

They breed scent hounds, and you can't call them dogs. No, they are foxhounds. They breed them to chase foxes, even though in the hunt I regularly participate in, it is not actually a fox. Instead they take the urine of a fox and spread it on the field prior to the hounds and horses being released. That is called a drag, and the hunt itself, a drag hunt. NO animals are harmed.

Drag hunting is conducted in a manner similar to foxhunting, with a field of mounted riders following a pack of foxhounds hunting the trail of a planted scent. The primary difference between foxhunting and drag hunting is the hounds are trained to hunt a prepared scent trail laid by a person dragging a material soaked in linseed/urine or another strong smelling substance.

A drag hunt course follows a predetermined route over jumps and obstacles. The scent, or line, is laid ten to thirty minutes prior to beginning the hunt. There are usually three to four lines of approximately 2 mi (3.2 km) each, laid for a day of hunting.

And so, there you are. Everybody is dressed formally (I just love that part—the formal dress with helmets on.) And all of a sudden, the master of the hounds comes out. All riders must face the master. He walks with the hounds, and then they are let loose, and then the riders follow. Off we go to chase the "fox"!

There are many obstacles during the hunt. Jumps, logs, trees, zigzag trails, mud, water, high jumps, low jumps, hidden water just beyond the jumps. There are usually ten to forty people riding at one time, facing a lot of different challenges. First field jumps and rides the fastest. Second field rides at a slower pace and does some jumps. Third field walks or trots with no jumps. It depends on what the rider is comfortable handling. And your horse's age has a lot to do with your chosen field. It is an exhilarating and thrilling feeling every time I ride.

(cont'd, Close Loop)

Horses in My Life—for Life

One of the times I was on my horse fox/drag hunting, a freaky accident happened. The hoof of my horse got caught in a hole, a very small hole, causing his leg to buckle. I lost my balance in the saddle, and fell off the horse to the hard ground with my knee still bent—hitting the ground with my bent knee. It was quite a high fall. I learned later my entire femur was shattered, and I will say it was probably the worst pain I've ever experienced.

I had to be air-lifted out of there, and it seemed like a lifetime before they could get to me. We were in the middle of a field, and it was not a pretty day. The weather was far from ideal, and it was hard just to see through the trees. It was quite an ordeal.

There I was at age fifty-nine, after my second major accident, back in the hospital—getting my leg repaired, coming out, recovering, learning to walk again, having to be lifted up on an air machine to even be able to stand. It was like the machinery they use to help a person who becomes paraplegic, where the machinery walks for you. I was off my feet in a wheelchair for two months. But I had a lot of help, and eventually, I was able to bear weight with the good trainers and coaches who guided me through my therapy. I had to step up, and up again to a second step, and back down. Up and down the steps, over and over, and eventually, I found myself putting my leg over the back of my horse, sitting up there, and yes, riding again.

After my accident, I couldn't walk let alone ride a horse. Even so, I did not ignore my horse and simply not show up at the barn. I still went there—I took a medical van so I could be lowered down to the stall in my wheelchair. I went there on crutches. I went there on a walker. I went there on a cane. And then, I could simply walk in to see my horse.

It was a good eight or nine months before I could get on a horse again. Was I nervous that first time back? Yes. But not like I was frightened to get back on. I was just apprehensive. The sadness of the possibility of never being able to ride again was too overwhelming for me. I thank God that fear dissipated. It proved unwarranted. I found myself back on my horse and able to ride, eventually, becoming good enough to hunt once again.

I feel young when I am on my horse. I think a lot of people share that feeling because you have to be athletic to handle these beasts. It is not for the ill-suited or people who are not in good shape. So again, it is back to being about taking care of yourself and staying healthy. If you want to be able to ride, that is what you need to do, and that being said, you also need to have a good horse.

My horse's name is On the Marc, and he is a great horse. He is highly trained. I found him in Upper Peninsula, Michigan, and he's been my buddy for about fifteen years now. I think the smartest thing a parent can do is to lease a horse for their child. This genuinely gives a child a good sense of responsibility, something to take care of with the brushing, cleaning, clipping, and shining them up, as well as showing up on time for classes. I've seen wonderful things happen with children who started and stayed with riding, and when they were adults, they were just different in a good way from people who don't have that interest.

A horse brings out the child in you. And I've heard that from other riders as well. Who doesn't love a horse? It is such a good feeling. At one time, I had up to four horses. Then I got down to two. You can only ride one at a time, so the pressure of having that many horses and trying to ride them all was a little too much. So now, I have only "Marc," whom I love. He's been my pal and companion through many challenges in my life. I hope he lasts forever.

CHAPTER 11

A COVID-19 Life

S ometime in the early part of this year (2020), I started thinking about planning an extravagant celebration for my 75th birthday. I rented a theater, a beautiful theater. I contracted several celebrities to perform, music artists in the industry. I was even planning to sit in on a set of music and surprise my guests by singing a few songs. Some of my friends aren't even aware that I do that, so it would have been quite a surprise. So much planning went into this, and then of course, the COVID-19 bomb hit. And that was that. It was the end of all that lovely planning.

Well, it would've been nice to have that celebration happen, but it's just a party. Compared to the seriousness of the horrible virus that hit home in many ways, a party is just not important. Several friends from New York and some close girlfriends in Chicago contracted COVID-19. I had been on a ski trip in early March with about twenty people when it hit. It was pretty much at the beginning of it, and several people on that trip came down with this virus. I myself cut my trip short, but some of the people who stayed on caught it.

Even so, I didn't comprehend the vast implications of the pandemic until they started closing down huge venues like Broadway, concerts, the NBA, air travel, summer activities, and on and on. Every year around the time of my birthday, I would celebrate by going to NYC for the Tony Awards and to Belmont to watch the horses, which I love. Everything was canceled.

So what else could I add to that? Well, I learned I needed hip replacement surgery. I swear, you could have knocked me down with a feather. I had no idea of needing such a drastic remedy to the pains I'd been having. A lot of pain in my back, my leg, my groin, but not my hip. I had been trying to consult a doctor, but none of them would see me. None of the hospitals would let you in unless you'd been diagnosed with the virus and needed hospitalization for that. It was a mess. But my dear husband got on the phone with some of his doctor friends, very insistent for them to see me. Finally, around that time, virtual meetings started taking place with doctors. I had managed to get X-rays taken at an urgent care walk-in clinic, and got them sent to the hospital for their records. The doctor took one look at them and said, "Well, at a glance, I can tell you this. You need a new hip. Your hip is totally gone."

"Okay," I said, after letting that sink in. "So, when should we fix this?"

And he said, "That is going to take some time."

"How much time? I haven't slept in four or five weeks." I had been in very bad pain, serious pain. I couldn't lie on my left side, my right side, my back. I slept in fits, and it was just a tough time.

"Well, I'm sorry," he said, "But we're looking at about three months."

I must have had a look of horror on my face. He added, "I'm sorry. All the procedures at the hospital have been halted until further notice. The only procedures that are going to be done right now are for life-threatening situations." Needless to say, I was pretty distraught.

But here again, I took a negative situation and turned it into a positive one. During the lockdown, I decided to use my time wisely. At Suzanne's suggestion, we jump-started the conception of this book together, which gave me the creative outlet I needed. It helped me through this period of COVID-19, and it continues to help me.

At-Home Facial Steps

At this point, almost everyone misses their beauty professionals and a well-deserved day at the spa. You might have been wondering how long you would have to wait without these sessions to keep you glowing from week to week. The good news is, you don't have to wait long at all.

While staying at home and maintaining social distancing drags on, no rule says you have to neglect the care and love your skin desperately needs. You can get all that glow and pampering from an at-home facial performed with your own tender hands. The trick is to have fun with it and savor every moment.

Here are the steps for a spa-worthy facial treatment at home.

1. **Cleanse**

   Cleansing is the hallmark of all things facial and skincare. You must ensure your skin is washed clean to rid it of oil residue, dirt, makeup, and other impurities. To cleanse, you can wipe off any makeup you have on with cleansing wipes. Then use an oil-based cleanser such as coconut oil or olive oil to wipe off most dirt. Finish with a mild foam cleanser and wash with lukewarm water.

2. **Exfoliate**

   Exfoliation is where the magic starts to remove dead skin cells and brighten your skin. When doing facials at home, you can choose between natural ingredients in your kitchen or formula scrubs. Homemade scrubs can be sugar, salt, or oatmeal scrubs. Rub the scrub into your face in a circular motion and rinse off after with lukewarm water.

3. **Massage**

   Now it's time to improve muscle tone and increase blood circulation for firmer and brighter skin. Taking a small amount of face massage cream or your favorite oil in your fingers massage the face from the middle of your forehead working toward your temples. Work in a gentle upward direction for the entire face. Do this for 10 minutes and rinse with water.

4. Steam

Open up your pores and prepare your skin to absorb beauty products with the steaming step. For this facial treatment, at-home steaming is as simple as boiling clean water in a pot and leaning over it when the stove is off. Let the steam caress your face for 5 to 10 minutes.

5. Masque

The masque you choose for your at-home facial depends on what your skin needs. You can use a hydrating cream masque, depuffing sheet masques for the eyes, or even an oil-absorbing clay masque. Again, you can look to your kitchen for a natural masque such as an oatmeal and avocado blend.

Leave the masque on for up to 15 minutes before washing off.

The last step is to moisturize and massage. Get your favorite serum and moisturizer and layer them both on in gentle upward motions.

Wearing a Mask Provides This Anti-Aging Benefit

It's no longer news that wearing face masks or any form of face shield is the new normal. Masks such as surgical face masks made from layers of cotton, face shields, and so on are a major part of the personal protective equipment (PPE) designed to enhance protection and reduce or prevent the spread of the virus.

At first, wearing a mask daily was like ruining a party for most beauty and fashion lovers. But in recent times, people are starting to adapt and find new ways to incorporate the face-covering with their style.

Some exciting news is the discovery that wearing a mask can also provide anti-aging benefits. Experts and extensive mask users have confirmed this benefit, and it's almost easy to see how wearing a mask regularly can contribute to anti-aging. Dermatologists will tell you that anything that offers skin coverage adds a layer of protection from the sun.

Why is this important and how does it work? Get all the facts straight below.

How the Sun Contributes to Aging

None of us can escape getting older, and as the aging process progresses, the signs will start to show. When it comes to intrinsic or chronological aging, we have no way of controlling it. But with external factors that contribute to or speed up signs of aging, we can exercise control to reduce or eliminate their effects.

One such external factor is the sun. Did you know that an entire 90 percent of skin aging can be blamed on the sun? The effects of ultraviolet (UV) rays on the skin and the aging process include the reduction of proteins or breakdown of collagen in the skin that ultimately leads to a loss of youthful appearance over a long time. UV radiation also causes aging by exacerbating the development of wrinkles, age spots, and hyperpigmentation on the skin.

The best way to avoid or reduce the effects of the sun on the skin is to prevent exposure or use sun protection. Wearing the proper clothing is one way to protect the skin from UV radiation just like using sunscreen helps too.

Face masks are made of materials that block or reduce exposure to UV radiation, just like your regular clothing. Having them on consistently when outdoors helps your skin stay protected, hydrated, and vibrant.

But you should also note . . .

While wearing a face mask offers you anti-aging benefits as a layer of protection from the sun, you shouldn't hold back on applying sunscreen. Since the mask can wipe off your sunscreen and any materials applied on the face, it's important to reapply a few times in a day when you take the mask off. Using sunscreen is especially important for those spending long hours outdoors, and necessary to prevent the not-so-pretty sight of tan lines.

If you also have skin problems such as acne and eczema, taking measures to prevent flare-ups due to the face covering is just as relevant as claiming the anti-aging benefits.

Lipstick Index vs. Mascara Index

A brief history lesson will enable us to understand the relevance or meaning of the lipstick index.

In the early 2000s, Leonard Lauder, chairman of the board of Estee Lauder, coined the term the *lipstick index* and described it as an economic indicator. He described that purchases of cosmetics, especially lipsticks, were related to economic health. The idea or opinion behind this was that during economic distress women ditch other luxury items like clothes and shoes and replace them with lipsticks.

As interesting as this may sound, the reality is that lipstick sales have also experienced growth during increased economic activity. Hence, this claim has been discredited.

Regardless, the lipstick index remains an indicator of consumer trends and behaviors. Companies use it to assess consumer confidence. In the case of the coronavirus, the lipstick index might indicate more than the economic recession and pave the way for what is now being called the *mascara index*.

With people now able to leave their homes, makeup will return to the scene with a new demand but rather than a demand for lipstick, we may see high demands for mascara and other eye makeup items. Chris Ventry, a Vice President of the Consumer and Retail Practice of management consultancy SSA & Company, states it clearly, "As more and more people are wearing masks, they're emphasizing other forms of makeup. People might get very creative with how they accessorize their eyes."

If your mouth must be covered, then the next best way to treat yourself to a daily luxury is to focus on the eyes. This will include thick, glossy, and ultra-black mascara that makes your eyes more outstanding and "battable." Eyeliners and eye makeup colors that match masks may also be the new normal.

Already, CNN reported that Alibaba has seen a 150 percent increase in sales of eye cosmetics since mid-February. Some YouTubers and beauty enthusiasts have already taken to the screens and social media to present mask makeup clips. You can certainly say it's that time to experiment which colors enhance your iris and just make the eyes pop. Product developers should get a head start now, working double time on everything from eye shadow palettes to eyeliners.

While much is still unclear, we have to be prepared, right? In the end, the situation with the coronavirus or maybe the availability of a vaccine can determine whether the lipstick index will win out over its growing counterpart.

Looking Forward

I finally did get my surgery when the writing of this book was in full swing, which was unbelievable. I was in the hospital for two days, and I think many of my friends were somewhat fearful that I should go into the hospital because they were caring for so many coronavirus patients at that time. But I was never really frightened of that. Northwestern Hospital, where I had the surgery, knows very well how to take care of everything. They have certain wings for keeping the virus contained, and everything was clean, clean, clean. I never had a moment of fear in that regard the whole time I was there. It was all handled properly. I had a huge room, away from anyone, and everyone wore masks. I had the surgery, and I am so happy that I did.

I am looking forward to the time when the world comes back to some normality, and I can start doing the things I love, once again, such as traveling internationally. I have started to travel domestically – my first post-lockdown destination was Aspen, where Arny and I got to visit with Jill St. John and Robert Wagner at their home – it was a great time. Thank you, Jill & RJ!

I don't think we'll see the world back to normal as we knew it for some time. But remember one thing: the longest road starts with the first step.

Conclusion

We have covered some essential topics in the course of this book—keeping the faith, maintaining determination, regaining confidence, handling drama, practicing good habits that will help you keep and maintain your youth, and facing fears. These are all important things to be addressed for one's life to be happy. That sounds like a handful, but frankly, life is a handful. There are no real silver spoons, and even if someone has something like that to rely on, life is still tough.

Having the strength to stay confident in spite of whatever happens to be going on in life and continuing to replace negativity with positivity is truly a challenge. It is far from being an easy task, but no one said life would be easy. And never forget that the joy comes in the course of the journey itself. In fact, the joy is all in the journey, not in the destination. And why is that? Because for most of us humans, when we arrive at that desired destination, it's not what we expected. It is just not enough. People are never happy with that. That is the reason you need to make the journey itself as fulfilling as possible, and most people don't seem to know this.

I could give you several examples of some friends— authors, artists, talented celebrities— who were trying to climb to the top. They fought their way, scratching and clawing, whatever they had to do even if it would have meant stepping over their own mother, all to get to the top.

What is that top? What exactly does *the top* mean? Where does it say that the top is going to equal happiness? Frankly, in most cases, it doesn't. Why not? Because the top is quite a disappointment. I have asked people over and over again this big question because it has always been a question mark in my own mind: "So, how does it feel to be up there and successful?" And so many times, they have answered that when they got there, they asked themselves, "Is this all there is? Really, this is it?" There is a good lesson to be learned from that. And so, I learned it.

I am a goal-oriented person, and I keep on reinventing myself, I know I may never be satisfied, and perhaps, I never want to be. This is the trait of an artist. I want to always keep trying new things because that is the fun of it. As soon as I have accomplished something, I realize "That's it," and I'm on to something else. Now, why is that? Because, as humans, we're seldom satisfied. That's just one of those built-in faults God gave us.

When I shattered my femur and was thinking horrible thoughts like I'd never be able to ride again, if instead of working hard and getting back on my horse by taking all that negativity, all that self-doubt and transforming it into positive energy, what if I'd given up hope? I'd have never been on my horse again. It is all about accepting change because throughout our entire life, nothing stays the same. Everything is always evolving. It is always changing. And so, that is why I encourage people—readers, friends, family— to practice habits that will give them the strength and confidence to do that.

As we get older, our memory just isn't the same as it was. Cognition often declines in our brain, which is a part of aging. So don't feel badly about that. Embrace it, if you can, and do something about it.

I kept on practicing it, using repetition and dedication, and more repetition. And over time, I developed my muscle memory, just like an athlete develops physical muscle. An athlete is not an athlete because he or she works out or practices once a week with the team or in the field or lifts weights. This is something you have to do all the time or it doesn't work. Same thing with your muscle memory— repetition, dedication, discipline.

Plus, you'll never be bored if you do this. I get frustrated when I hear people say, "I'm so bored. Look at this horrible virus situation everybody's in. We have nothing to do." That's insane because there are plenty of things you can do to improve yourself. Take up a little sport in your house, take up the piano, adopt a dog—plant some seeds and they'll grow. You just need to get off your butt and do something. Plan something. If you don't water a plant, it dies. Same thing with our bodies. Same thing with our minds.

I tend to strive for perfection, even though I know I probably will never get there. But at least it gives me an outlet to try and create something, do something. And that is my point—you need to find something to do. Here I am, just having turned 75 years old. Yikes! Hold onto your helmet. It's like I have this vision of myself as if I were peeking from behind a door, and I have to ask, "Who is that girl? Could that be me? Am I really 75 years old? No, no, no, that can't be me. I don't want to be 75. I want to be 25, 35, 45." But that is not possible. I've had to either accept my age or look foolish trying to look younger than I was in the public's eye, and more importantly, to myself. Clinging to your youth just doesn't work.

I have been fortunate in that I was born with some pretty good genes, and certainly, that has helped me over my entire life. By facing my age and not just to myself, but essentially announcing it and letting it out there, I was faced with a lot of criticism. I took a risk because a lot of my work depended on people thinking I was much younger. Even some friends thought, "Well, she's too old to hang out with us. We don't have anything in common." But the truth is, once I get out on the dance floor, I can out dance most of them. I could do a lot of things most of my friends could not do, and they are half my age. So that never stops me. But I was pretty worried about putting my age out there like that. I was uncomfortable, and still am a little. Let me tell you, it was not easy. But it is what it is.

So this is what I decided to do to help me with that. Instead of hiding my age, I decided to embrace it and throw myself a huge party. I invited over 300 people to come celebrate my 75th birthday, out in the public with tons of friends, publicity, cameras, newspapers, some celebrities—you name it. I rented a big theater, and that was where I was going to have my big bash. Everything was planned over several months. And then bang, COVID-19 hits, and the world shuts down. That was the end of my celebration.

So of course, we're all in our houses for a while, for a long time, actually. And some of us have taken this time to think. Some of us just furiously ran around the household, cleaning the closets, baking cakes (after running and getting the flour), cleaning our desk, rearranging the cabinets, you name it. But for me, I wanted to think. I wanted to use my brain and think about this. And I've had so much time to do this. What I started to feel was that what's really important to me is fresh air, good friends, family, nature, animals, feel-good stuff. Not all that craziness that is going on in the outer world.

I am a social creature, and I like a party just like the next person. But frankly, it doesn't mean as much as it used to. I, along with a lot of other people in the world, took a lot for granted. Maybe it was time for a higher power, a Supreme being, to come down and say, "Okay, we're going to take a few of these pleasures away."

I have always been thankful, and now I am even more so. Just thinking about that and feeling it and being in the present moment was sort of a gift to myself.

My wish for all my readers would be to continue to love and never stop dreaming. Always surround yourself with beauty, peace, carefreeness, and love. And though I did not include this in my beauty tips earlier in this book, this is how I truly feel—one of the best beauty tips of all is to fall in love. That is the best beauty treatment you could ever have.

So all that being said, I would like to thank those of you who have helped me through this journey, and continue to do so even today: my rock, loyal, and dedicated husband, Arny Granat; my most loyal friend and business partner, Suzanne Tripaldi; and a special thanks to Rob Kosberg and the BSP team. I could not have done it without all of you. God bless.

50 is the BEGINNING, not the END

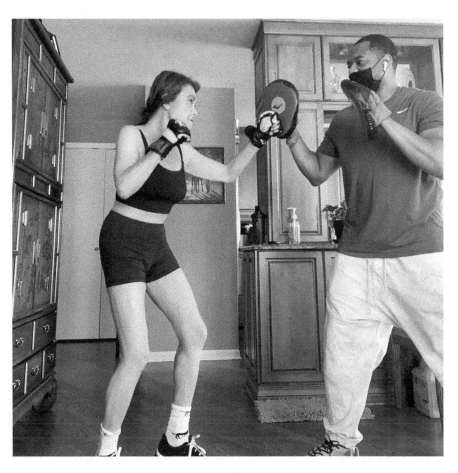

Beating Father Time

About
Irene Michaels

Irene Michaels is a lifelong entertainer, entrepreneur, and accomplished equestrian, who has made it a priority to lead an active and healthy lifestyle. She discovered her passion for dance at the age of eleven and went on to a career as a dancer, model, actress, owner of a successful modeling agency, and producer. She is widely recognized as a beauty and luxury lifestyle expert. Since 2008, her popular website, I On the Scene, has continued to share the full scoop on entertainment, culture, and fashion to readers worldwide. Released under her signature brand, I On Youth Collection by Irene Michaels™ Roll-On Serum filled a need for a convenient, moderately priced, and effective anti-aging skincare product. An avid animal lover, Irene earned her Colors, a great honor in the equestrian community, enabling her to ride in prestigious hunts globally. Irene lives with her husband, Arny Granat, in her hometown, Chicago.

CPSIA information can be obtained
at www.ICGtesting.com
Printed in the USA
BVHW041146240521
608005BV00002B/6